PRAISE FOR
HEALING HABITS

"*Healing Habits* isn't a quick fix . . . but rather, a lasting one. Rebecca Renck shows us how to unravel the roots and triggers of illness, shaping new strategies for healthier living. She speaks from the personal understanding of meeting health challenges, and insight fashioned from a deeper truth."

–Donna DeNomme, award-winning, internationally published author *8 Keys to Wholeness: Tools for Hope-Filled Healing*

"Rebecca Renck's journey is a powerful testament to courage and resilience. With grace and determination, she empowers us with lifestyle strategies to create vibrant health. Her wisdom is born from personal experience and a deep understanding of the body's innate ability to heal."

–Dr. Veronique Desaulniers DC, Founder of *Breast Cancer Conqueror* and *The 7 Essentials*

HEALING HABITS

HEALING HABITS

How to Help Your Body Heal Itself from Chronic Illness

REBECCA RENCK

© Rebecca Renck Copyright 2025

All rights reserved. No part of this book may be used or reproduced by any means, graphic, electronic, or mechanical, including photocopying, recording, taping or by any other information storage retrieval system without the written permission of the author except in the case of brief quotations embodied in critical articles and reviews.

Because of the dynamic nature of the internet, any web addresses or links contained in this book may have changed since publication and may no longer be valid. The views expressed in this work are solely those of the author.

The author of this book does not profess to be a certified medical practitioner or dispense medical advice or prescribe the use of any technique as a form of treatment for physical, emotional, or medical problems in lieu of the advice of a physician, either directly or indirectly. The intent of the author is only to offer information of a general nature to help you in your quest for emotional and spiritual well-being. In the event you use any of the information in this book for yourself, which is your constitutional right, the author and the publisher assume no responsibility for your actions.

Any people depicted in stock imagery are models, and such images are being used for illustrative purposes only.

Print information available on the last page.

ISBN (paperback): 979-8-89686-198-0
ISBN (ebook): 979-8-89686-189-8
ISBN (Audible): 979-8-89686-196-6

Book design and production by www.AuthorSuccess.com

Printed in the United States of America

I dedicate this book to my father who passed away when I was writing this. He was a master stone mason by trade and helped me to understand the importance of building a strong foundation of family, of love, and of health.

Contents

Foreword	xi
Introduction	1
Building a Foundation	3
CHAPTER 1: A Disease Arrived On My Doorstep	7
CHAPTER 2: What Does It Take To Help a Body Heal Itself?	13
Take Responsibility	15
You Are Never Past the Point of No Return	16
Get Down and Dirty With the Root Causes of the Dis-Ease	17
Provide the Correct Environment	19
CHAPTER 3: A PRODUCT OF YOUR HABITS	21
Changing Behaviors	22
An Empowered Identity	23
Moment To Moment: Compounding Small Habits	25
How Do You Make It Stick?	27
CHAPTER 4: HOW TO USE THIS BOOK	31
The Breaking Point	31
Your Future Self	32
PRINCIPLES AND HABITS	37
PRINCIPLE 1: The Decision—This Is Your Game Now	39
Trust Yourself to Take Care of You	40
PRINCIPLE 2: YOUR REASON WHY	47
Deciding What and Why	49
Who You Are At Your Core	50
PRINCIPLE 3: HARNESSING YOUR FAITH	57
Faith In Your Body	58
Finding Strength	59
PRINCIPLE 4: THE HAWK'S EYE PERSPECTIVE	63
Emotional Guidance System	64

PRINCIPLE 5: TURN 180 DEGREES	**71**
The Courage to Change	72
PRINCIPLE 6: STANDARD PROTOCOL	**79**
Only Treating the Symptom	80
PRINCIPLE 7: DETOX YOUR ENVIRONMENT	**87**
Environmental Pollutants	88
Emotional Toxins	88
PRINCIPLE 8: DIET AND NUTRITION	**93**
The 'Normal' Standard American Diet (Sad)	95
PRINCIPLE 9: GRATITUDE AND GRACE	**103**
Giving Yourself Grace	105
PRINCIPLE 10: TIME WELL SPENT	**109**
Obligations	111
Aims and Desires	112
Shoulds	113
PRINCIPLE 11: A BODY IN MOTION	**119**
The Gym of Life	120
PRINCIPLE 12: SETTING BOUNDARIES	**123**
Lifestyle Enhancers	124
Following the Crowd	125
The Absolute Nos	127
The Absolute Yesses	128
PRINCIPLE 13: CRAVINGS, IMPULSES, AND ADDICTIONS	**131**
Redirecting Your Focus	133
PRINCIPLE 14: THE LAW OF ATTRACTION	**137**
The Power of Goodwill	138
PRINCIPLE 15: ROUTINES AND RHYTHMS	**142**
Intuitive Patterns	144
PRINCIPLE 16: HEALING SPACES	**149**
Nature as Healer	151
Clearing the Inside Clutter	152

PRINCIPLE 17 :	MAKE IT SIMPLE	158
	Complexity of Our Modern Life	159
PRINCIPLE 18 :	CREATIVE COMFORT	164
	The Artist Within	165
PRINCIPLE 19:	REFLECT AND EVALUATE	169
	Some Things Work, Some Don't	171
PRINCIPLE 20:	PUT A SMILE ON IT	176
	Happy As a Lark	177
CONCLUSION:	THRIVING NOT JUST SURVIVING	181
	Life Beyond Illness	184
CITATIONS		186
RESOURCES		187
ACKNOWLEDGMENTS		190

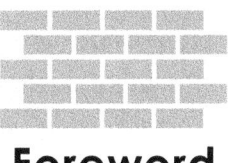

Foreword

While the idea of *you* being the most valuable player (MVP) on your collaborative medical team for dealing with your chronic illness may seem a bit outlandish or a bit of a stretch at first, it is important to understand the historical foundations of Hermetic medicine which was taught to me in medical school, as it still is today to all first-year medical students. Then, at the end of our training, all new physicians take some form of the Hippocratic Oath to uphold certain ethical standards based on the teachings of the Greek physician Hippocrates (460-370 BC), including the principles of medical confidentiality and to "at least do no harm."

However, Imhotep (2686-2613 BC) is considered to be the 'father of medicine' in ancient Egypt, preceding Hippocrates by thousands of years. He practiced a comprehensive approach, treating diseases holistically and integrating surgery, herbal medicine, and spiritual healing. The Greek and Egyptian traditions merged, influencing Western medicine, but over time, medicine shifted and became increasingly materialistic and separated from its holistic spiritual and philosophical elements.

THE SHIFT AWAY FROM HOLISTIC HEALING

In the fifth century BC, Hippocrates introduced a more scientific, materialistic approach, which led to the separation of medicine from philosophy and spirituality. Modern medicine, influenced by this shift, became physically symptom-focused and fragmented into specialties, often neglecting the emotional, mental, and spiritual aspects of health. It was a German-Swiss physician named Paracelsus (1493—1541) who pioneered the use of minerals and other chemicals in medicine. However, he also sought to restore ancient healing wisdom, emphasizing the Hermetic principles that viewed disease as influenced by spiritual, mental, and cosmic factors.

HERMETIC CAUSES AND CURES FOR DISEASE

The principles and practices of Hermetic medicine are based on the teachings of the ancient Egyptian god Thoth and the Greek god Hermes. Despite modern skepticism, Hermetic healing principles remain foundational in medical history and are still studied in medical schools.

The teachings state that the seven causes of disease include: spiritual imbalances, karma, astrological influences, emotional disharmonies, unhealthy mental attitudes, overtaxing the physical body, and external toxins.

The seven Hermetic cures include: invocations, energy healing (vibrations, color, sound therapy), talismans, herbal remedies, prayer, preventative lifestyle measures, and practical physical medical interventions.

THE NEED FOR HOLISTIC MEDICAL EDUCATION AND APPROACHES

Modern medicine has made heroic leaps in advancing physical investigation and approaches to disease processes. The advances in surgical techniques and modern diagnostic tools such as MRIs and CT scans have led to an almost magical ability to diagnose issues that would have been hidden from our view before such technologies existed. These approaches have saved many lives in emergency situations. However, modern medicine has widely been focused on treatment of disease that is already present rather than a wellness focus.

Modern medical training focuses on physical diagnosis and pharmacological treatment but lacks meaningful education on nutrition, alternative healing methods, and mind-body connections. The future of medicine should integrate traditional courses with teachings on energy medicine, herbal and homeopathic remedies, spiritual anatomy, sound/color healing, and the metaphysical wisdom that has been available to us since the time of Imhotep.

A VISION FOR THE FUTURE OF MEDICINE

Physicians should be trained not only in scientific knowledge but also as healers with awareness of the body, mind, and spirit and a focus on preventative wellness rather than on disease states. All people should be empowered and educated in the importance of their own choices and options toward creating a path to enhancing wellness and vitality rather than a slippery slope toward disease and illness.

Modern medicine must reclaim its holistic roots, blending scientific advancements with ancient healing wisdom. This transformation would create a more complete and compassionate healthcare system, empowering physicians and patients alike. Healing should be based on achieving and maintaining a high vibrational state, fostering deep connections between doctor and patient, and promoting true wellness rather than mere disease management.

PRAISE FOR THE BRAVE WORK OF REBECCA RENCK

I have used holistic integrative (mind/body/emotion/spirit) approaches in my thirty-five years of clinical psychiatric practice and over twenty years of teaching classes on healing and personal transformation. I have personally used the approaches that I have taught and that Rebecca Renck espouses in her latest work: *Healing Habits: How to Help Your Body Heal Itself from Chronic Illness*. I have seen amazing shifts (emotionally, mentally, physically, and spiritually) in the thousands of people who I have taught, worked with, or coached over the past three decades . . . it works.

With love and holistic understanding, complete healing of the physical, emotional, and spiritual self becomes possible. I applaud Ms. Renck's bravery in sharing her own journey and for creating a meaningful, easy-to-understand and use handbook for others with chronic illness.

Thank you, Rebecca for being such a bright light to others in their journey!

Tracy Latz, M.D., M.S, Mh.D.
Co-author of *Bye-Bye Self-Sabotage:
Drop Your Baggage Love Your Life*
'Shift Doctor' at ShiftYourLIfe.com,
Shift Your Life TV Channel on YouTube

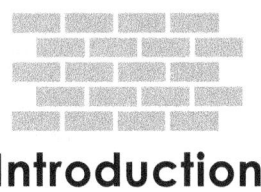

Introduction

The cruelest part of disease is not the pain it brings, but the way it steals tomorrow's promise.

Being diagnosed with a chronic illness is a hard blow in our lives. There is no good time to be sick. There is no good time to be unable to care for our loved ones or not participate fully in life's activities. There is no good time to feel like a victim of a disease, to live with debilitating or restrictive symptoms, or to have no one understand that the pain is NOT in your head but your body. And to make the blow even more on target, it usually comes when we are at our prime; at a time when things are going well in our lives: athletes rising to the top of their game, college students studying for their dream careers, entrepreneurs finally showing a profit, moms finding a rhythm in the daily busy-ness. Chronic illness can affect anyone at any time.

Chronic illnesses have a significant impact on the American population, with approximately 60 percent of adults living with at least one diagnosed condition, and 40 percent of those managing two or more. These illnesses include what are now common diseases such as heart disease, diabetes, arthritis, mental health disorders, and over eighty types of autoimmune diseases. Chronic illness is the leading cause of death and disability in the US and contributes to 75 percent of the nation's healthcare spending. The healthcare industry, including the cost of medical treatments, medications, insurance, and the sheer numbers of patients put a strain not only on the country's economics, but personal finances as well. These disheartening truths point to a chronically ill society that has been created in less than sixty years.

> **Isn't it frustrating that even with all the 'advancements' in medicine, as a society we are sicker than ever?**

How did the health of our bodies become an industry with a significant portion of our nation's economy (personal and government) struggling with or, in some cases, profiting from pharmaceutical, insurance, and medical care? When and why did medical health care transmute into disease care? With all the advances in medical science, why are these diseases becoming increasingly prevalent to the point of being considered common?

There are exceptions due to genetic predispositions or injuries, and I am not downplaying or referring to those situations in any way, but for the average person who is diagnosed with a disease with no other qualifiers, we must ask ourselves: how did we get to this point? Is Western conventional medicine failing us, or are we failing ourselves by how we take care of our bodies? Are our culture, foods, and lifestyle literally making us sick?

Chronic disease can be defined as a long-lasting condition that persists for a year or more, requires ongoing medical attention or limits activities of daily living, and can be managed but not cured. These illnesses often result from a combination of genetic, environmental, and lifestyle factors, and they affect multiple body systems requiring continuous care and management.

Chronic illnesses develop in our bodies over time; they are not caught like a cold, nor do they typically stem directly from infection or viruses. By the time symptoms are severe enough to garner our attention, the illness is usually in full rampage. The body has been stressed enough in some way, shape, or form by a root cause that it can no longer function as it was meant to, and this leads to the chronic symptoms experienced.

The human body is an intricate and interconnected system where every organ, tissue, and cell play a vital role in maintaining overall health and function rather than operating as isolated parts. This holistic perspective emphasizes that healing and well-being rely on looking at the body as a whole, rather than focusing solely on individual symptoms or areas.

If we combine the thoughts that the body has the ability to heal itself and is a complex interconnected system that has been overwhelmed by outside factors, common sense leads me to believe that by identifying and addressing the root causes, a chronically ill body has a good chance to heal.

We have all seen evidence of the natural ability to heal from a cut, a broken bone, a cold virus, or from infection without much intervention. There are also tens of thousands of examples of those who reversed cancer, overcame disabilities, and successfully managed chronic illnesses. Giving the body a chance to heal is not only possible but doable.

□ □ □

BUILDING A FOUNDATION

I am disheartened by the amount of disease I see today, and you should be too. The over-reliance on medications and surgeries thrown at a patient for treatment without cause or outcome is unacceptable, and the best thing we can do for ourselves is to take our health into our own hands. By demanding to know the reason why you feel like hell, you will start asking questions, and with questions come answers.

Conventional medicine may have very few answers to offer you. However, if you ask these questions of yourself and of your own body, you will get some very useful information. Your body, through conscious intuition, can tell you how the things we unknowingly or (by throwing caution to the wind) knowingly do in our daily life, such as what toxins we expose ourselves to, what we eat, and stress over, all can be root causes of our problem. By questioning your current habits and consciously acknowledging what and why you do what you do, you receive not only some usable answers but also a starting point. To receive a different outcome, you need to do something different, and the exciting part is that each day offers a fresh start. You have the opportunity to do something, everything, or nothing different each day that will either support or continue to harm your body. The choice is yours.

This book is about how you can tap into that natural healing ability to your advantage. To embrace the belief that the body can heal itself, you only need to provide the correct environment; the body will take care of the rest. The environment that helps the body heal can look different for each of us, but there are some basic similarities, which I share with you here. I want to make the argument that no matter where you are starting from today, with awareness, knowledge, and healthier lifestyle habits, it is within anyone's capability to accomplish good health. The following pages describe the principles and habits I stumbled into over the last thirty-four years that I have found supported my disease (health) management and helped my body to heal itself. There are no outlandish ideas or new-fangled therapies, just things many of us do each day that, when given the proper twist of perspective and attention, can be used to our advantage.

Managing my chronic illnesses, I developed a lifestyle that supported feeling good and reduced not only the symptoms, but also the amount of disease in my body. This was accomplished with minimal medical intervention and certainly without the full blanket of standard medical protocol routinely prescribed.

My story may seem exceptional, but that is only because something inside me would not let me accept the situations I found myself in when presented with a disease and its prognosis. I am here to give you permission, hand you the tools, and then give an encouraging push for you to see that being diagnosed and then living with a chronic illness is not the dire ending we believe it to be. My solution was to understand what the symptoms were telling me, adjust my habits, and create a healing environment and sustainable lifestyle. While medical intervention is sometimes necessary, the reality is that chronic illnesses are better managed over time through lifestyle changes—an area where you hold the ultimate authority.

The book is structured into four chapters and twenty healing principles and habits. It begins with a basic overview of the essential aspects of a healthy lifestyle and emphasizes the importance of making conscious decisions. Each healing principle is paired with a practical healing habit, offering actionable examples and suggestions to help you transform your behaviors and build habits that promote sustainable good health. By embracing these principles with the right perspective and putting in a small amount of effort to develop new habits, you will find yourself on a journey to:

1. See improvement in your symptoms
2. Experience empowerment in self-care
3. Gain a practical tool set and roadmap for sustainable health, and
4. Help your body heal itself

This book is your guide to unlocking your body's natural healing potential, one habit at a time. By doing so, you can cultivate the mindset needed to understand that both your health and your lifestyle are shaped by your behaviors and habits.

◻ ◻ ◻

Healing as defined in this book is not a medical or scientific term. Rather, it's the body's natural ability to produce healthy cells that function optimally in their intended roles.

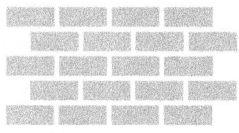

CHAPTER 1

A Disease Arrived On My Doorstep

I grew up in a healthy family during the sixties and seventies in the clear mountain air of Colorado, and by most standards had a good childhood. We ate home-cooked, well-rounded meals right off the food pyramid that circulated in the sixties and sparingly enjoyed the prepackaged, prepared frozen dinners that were all the rage at the time. I was involved in scouting, book clubs, and social groups.

When I was diagnosed with Crohn's disease at thirty, I had been happily married for nine years, had four young children, had lost a quarter of my normal body weight, and was so malnourished that walking up a short flight of stairs had me sitting and resting at the top. Eating an orange had me doubling over in pain, and VHS videos had become the babysitter of my young ones while I lay on the couch. Going out of the house to eat or participate in any activity was a cause of pain, embarrassment, or struggle. I had no idea how I had gotten to this point of ill health, only that my symptoms had worsened over several months to the point where I had to admit that something was not right.

I am not sure (after being misdiagnosed with rheumatoid arthritis and the flu) how I came across the female internal medicine doctor, but she put me in the hospital, did the correct tests, and finally diagnosed my malady as Crohn's disease. I remember her as somewhat of an angel. As most of the acute symptoms subsided, I was ecstatic in the prednisone drug-induced high,—thinking all my problems were solved and I was on the road to good health. I quickly realized the fallacy in the belief that feeling better equaled being healed when my angel doctor informed me that I had a chronic disease with no cure that would only get worse with time and included a probable surgery within five years.

Medications in 1990 were limited and I was allergic to two of them, leaving not much in the way of conventional medicine to manage my disease short of the promised surgery and some lifestyle changes. There was no book on what those lifestyle changes meant other than 'maybe it is the food you are eating.' Considering at the time I was not eating anything that didn't cause distress, that only fueled my frustration. As my heart sank lower and lower, I realized that my real issues with this disease had just begun.

I felt very lost, alone, and scared, but I see this now as the catalyst to how I was able to adopt an 'outside of the box' thinking. There were no real answers, so I needed to find some. A 'disease' came as a surprise to me, as I had never been exposed to anyone so chronically ill. I had no references, so I had no illusions about what conventional medicine could or could not do or even if I should follow the limited protocol available. Going to the doctor until then had consisted of prenatal and childcare appointments, all normal 'health care' related, and none requiring any lifelong management.

I was not a fan of the medication and its side effects or the surgery prognosis and soon found myself refusing to believe that those treatments were even a long-term option for me. Even with the pain and acute symptoms I was experiencing, an independent nature surfaced, and I made the decision that if the disease was manageable, I was going to try to manage it with as little medical intervention as possible. I was lucky to have the support of my 'angel doctor' who opened my eyes to the importance of taking care of myself with some alternative therapies, and honestly just looking outside that conventional medicine box. I had no idea how I was going to accomplish managing this illness or what it would look like over my lifetime, but I vowed to find a way and give it my best shot.

The path I ultimately followed was not wholly conventional or wholly holistic. There was no roadmap, and it certainly contained a lot of trial and error as I drew from a combination of the two modalities. But I can say that, just like most things in life, the end result has been well worth the struggle and well worth the effort. I am healthier today than I have ever been, and looking back, it was much less of a struggle than the treatments I have seen my fellow patients undergo.

> **I found a grace in taking care of myself that I did not know was missing. I found continued confidence in my intuition. I found strength in my mind and body that served me well, And I found the truth that when allowed, the body can heal itself.**

I wrote my first book in 2015, *Live Healthy with Crohn's Disease*, and during the writing phase, many of my symptoms suddenly flared up. Reliving the struggle, pain, shame, and personal resolve I had endured brought up so many emotions. I realized how much trauma I had been through and had yet to release. The book was therapeutic in that regard. I realized full force that I had lived much of my life keeping my illness a secret. Due to shame and fear, only my closest family and friends knew I had been diagnosed with a disease. The inner call to write and help others with my story was having a direct confrontation with that fear of trying not to be seen.

Within months of that time, I felt an intuitive nudge to have a mammogram and was diagnosed with breast cancer. As prevalent as cancer is, it was not something I had personally dealt with within my family sphere, and I was again thrust into an unknown world. After having the small tumor removed, I made the decision to refuse the eighteen months of 'preventative' drugs, chemo, and radiation prescribed by two oncologists and instead relied on the surgeon's evaluation that the cancer had been removed with the surgery. Having already managed a disease for over twenty-five years, and with a strong belief in the body being able to heal itself, I again summoned faith in and listened to my body. The realization hit me again of how much our buried emotional issues and day-to-day physical habits can play out as illness in our bodies. I pivoted, improved my lifestyle habits, looked at how I was showing up in my relationships, learned all I could about holistic cancer treatments and find myself, now over ten years later, still cancer free. I have not neglected scheduling routine check-ups and tests, and it has been gratifying to see that my healthy lifestyle habits have worked in so many instances.

I do not believe that my story is unique in having been diagnosed with these unfortunately common diseases. I do believe it is unique in how I managed them, my decisions made against the conventional norm and mindset, and belief in myself above all others. I still have Crohn's disease, and I still have cancer, but I refuse to let my identity be of a diseased victim, and I refuse to live my life in worry, pain, and suffering. I have weeks when I eat too much sugar, I have months where the role of caretaker and losing a family member robs me of sleep, I stress over money, and I cringe over the world we are leaving our grandchildren. I also eat well, am creative, enjoy my work, and love spending time with children, helping them to see the world with awe and wonder. I help, hope, and find glimmers everywhere I go. In short, I have developed an identity of balancing the stressful modern world we live in with taking care to supply my body with what it needs to thrive—both physically and emotionally.

If you are still breathing and if your heart is still beating, then you have the power of choice—the authority—in how you live and look at your life. We are not just the creators of our lives, but the architect. An 'architect' embodies not only the creative role but also the visionary, the builder, the collaborator, the planner, and the supervisor of their designs. You are the architect of your life. You can decide how sick you want to be.

◻◻◻

"When you let go of who you are,
you become who you might be."

—RUMI

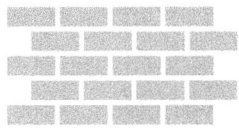

CHAPTER 2

What Does It Take To Help a Body Heal Itself?

The secret of health for both body and mind is to live in the present moment wisely and earnestly.

—BUDDHA

As commonplace as disease is in our society, it is still always a shock when you face a diagnosis yourself. And whether you are familiar with others who have chronic illnesses or, like in my case, you have no idea what to expect, it takes on a different level when it becomes personal. You may have felt something amiss in your own body for some time, or it may have come as a complete surprise. You may have been living with symptoms that came sporadically, then more frequently, and finally disrupting your life so dramatically that you had no option but to acknowledge and face the fear that something was terribly wrong.

No matter how your story has unfolded or where you find yourself, know that you are not alone, and others have been just where you are now. The diagnostic process of any chronic illness is often difficult, and it typically takes anywhere from six months to several years to receive a true diagnosis, and often with several misdiagnoses in between. Unfortunately, many go from doctor to doctor and have been ill for so long that pain and a low quality of life have become a normal, everyday struggle, and women especially, by this time, have multiple diseases flaring. If you have received an accurate diagnosis, you may now be excited and feel the worst is over much like I did. There is an answer, but over time, you begin to wonder what it truly means for you. What is the prognosis for a disease that doctors have identified but have no cure for? What does manageable really involve?

Life with a chronic illness is not easy, but it can be managed by reducing symptoms and allowing space for your body to heal. This book is about what 'managing' your disease takes. It is about what it means to release damaging habits to create space for new healing habits. It is about how to embody those habits into a healing lifestyle. It is about how to create an identity that sees you as the healthy person that supports your body to help heal itself. It is to remind you of the power you have over your life to be anything you want to be, and that includes being healthy and happy.

My experience of having controlled my Crohn's disease and then sustained a remission from breast cancer has led me to the awareness that choices I made in my daily life either helped reduce symptoms and supported healing or contributed to my illness, my symptoms, and my overall ill health. The sustainable healing choices all stemmed from healthy lifestyle habits that I developed over time. By taking responsibility for my health and by my willingness to make different choices, I was able to change the trajectory of disease in my body.

◻◻◻

TAKE RESPONSIBILITY

This is a call to take care of yourself, to take responsibility for youself. It is a call to denounce a total reliance on conventional Western medicine, its blanket protocols and disease management with only drugs and surgeries and instead work in tandem with your healthcare provider. (While medications and testing have their place, it is the reliance on only the medical system to manage your illness that needs to be addressed.) This current system of care does not see the body as an interconnected machine or as a whole person with a lifestyle and emotions and tends to treat just whatever particular symptom a person is experiencing. It is your job to not only get out of this conventional box but to identify, implement, and embody the healing that can be achieved on your own. This process is easier now than it has ever been. There is a flood of easily accessible information related to how the body works, alternative healing, plant medicine, energy modalities, or even how specific foods can help or hurt the body by causing inflammation. Helping the body to heal by using holistic alternatives in tandem with conventional Western medicine is not a new idea, but to make it all work for you, you must first take responsibility for your own health.

A responsibility to oneself is the first step in your personal disease management and is a two-part process. Step one is acknowledging that you have a hand in this disease that has developed in your body, and step two is understanding that you have the power to undo what has been done. As I mentioned before, most chronic illnesses develop in our bodies gradually over time, and given the right environment, the body has the ability to heal. (This may not be the case where there is permanent damage or surgeries to internal organs, but symptoms typically fall under this premise.) Your determined actions will make all the difference in your sustainable healing process. Be more concerned about where you are going from this day forward than where you have been.

In your healing journey, you will need to acknowledge where you are today and what got you here, to identify and admit what your role has been in the development of disease in your body, to look at your lifestyle, and to learn the ways to reverse the root causes.

You are the one in control, and good choices will have good results; continued bad choices will get you literally more symptoms; and more illness. In short, you can decide how sick and how much pain you want to be in. It is time to take responsibility and make some improvements for your own health and well-being.

If you are sick and tired of being sick and tired, take the leap of faith to follow a new path.

□□□

YOU ARE NEVER PAST THE POINT OF NO RETURN

Taking responsibility for your healing begins with accepting where you are today and acknowledging that your lifestyle has contributed to the problem. It is equally important to not beat yourself up over past decisions, whether made knowingly or unknowingly, and to recognize that there is always a path forward.

The bad news is that you have been diagnosed with a disease. The good news is no matter where you are in your diagnosis, you are not past the point of no return.

Your body is in a constant state of repair and renewal, ridding itself of dead cells and growing new cells each moment of each day. In fact, the human body produces over 3 million new cells per second to support, repair, and replace old, damaged cells. Cells are replacing areas of the body at varying speeds from a few seconds to days, and it is this remarkable regenerative capacity that gives credence to the idea that with the correct environment, the body can heal.

If no other factors change, diseased cells reproduce diseased cells, but when you can interrupt that process with supportive environments, you create conditions for healthy cells to thrive, which leads to healthy cells reproducing healthy cells. This holistic approach not only interrupts the cycle of disease but actively promotes healthy regeneration.

I believe all illnesses and diseases are a good thing in your life, a wake-up call, a blessing. A person could argue that any symptom outside perfect health is not a good thing, but you need to realize that blessings do not always have to feel good. Would you have taken action to stop the hectic pace or not eat processed foods before you got sick, knowing they were not good for you? Would you have changed your bad sleep habits for a good routine without a reason? Of course not, and that is okay. It is human nature to follow the norm and the path of least resistance. Be assured everyone has a disease—most people just don't know it yet.

□□□

GET DOWN AND DIRTY WITH THE ROOT CAUSES OF THE DIS-EASE

As you take responsibility for where you are today, you can begin to identify root causes. You can then learn what you need to learn and do what you need to do to eliminate these causes to create that healing environment. Every new piece of information and step forward helps to define a new normal lifestyle tailored just for you and will eventually lead to a sustainable remission. This requires an open mind, looking outside the box, trusting your instincts about things you are doing today, and a willingness to do things differently. It is an act of rebellion against the normal way of doing things, but one that will empower you.

Advanced research is now pointing to genetics and linking the gut microbiome as a root cause of many autoimmune diseases and chronic illnesses, but while an important piece, it isn't the complete answer. Treating a disease with only one focus isn't looking at the whole person or picture.

Habits and lifestyle include not only physical activity and symptoms but also the emotional, spiritual, and soulful essence of what makes you the person you are. If it is true that you are more than the sum of your physical parts, then so are the root causes of your illness. Common sense tells us there must be more than one reason the body went on a tirade.

A lifestyle is the culmination of the multitude of moments created by decisions, feelings, reactions, and habits. How we treat and feel about ourselves, deal with negativity, feed our cells, enjoy our time with others, the perception we have of our body, what we eat, when we rest, our purpose, and our values are just some examples of how interwoven the tapestry of our lives are. We are the sum of our parts energetically, and helping the body to heal itself means healing all of you. This is not about changing a few physical habits; it is seeing the root causes that conventional medicine seems to ignore, and those are about seeing the whole of you.

Each principle talks about physical and emotional aspects of life and how they relate to being a possible root cause. The ideas for habits to look at, change, improve on, or develop should also be looked in relation to how they apply to the whole of you. For instance, changing how you eat is not only about buying different groceries. You need to identify where the habits of what you eat come from: is it because you value convenience? Is it cultural? Do you hide behind foods or treat them as comfort? Is it a social prestige? The whys are just as important to identify as the whats.

As I became more aware of my habits, I knew without a doubt there were ways I was not taking the best care of myself. I believe that if you are here now, you also feel there are ways you could take better care of yourself and realize there is at least one habit or more that has become a root cause of the illness, and that it would help to eliminate such habits.

□□□

PROVIDE THE CORRECT ENVIRONMENT

It is often said that you become a reflection of the five people you spend the most time with. This concept can also be extended to the environment you surround and immerse yourself in. Just as the people closest to you influence your thoughts, habits, and behaviors, so too does your environment. The spaces you frequent, the energy of the communities around you, and even the information you read, hear, and speak all play a significant role in defining who you are. Developing a healing environment for our cells to regenerate and our body to function optimally needs to be done as a combination of our physical and emotional environment. To succeed in any area of change, your surroundings must align with your desired outcome. One without the other is less likely to create sustainable healing.

Our environment influences us as a framework that shapes our reactions. These reactions are often triggered by our surroundings, guiding us toward our next steps. For example, if you are trying to eat a healthier diet and your environment is filled with junk food—like chips on the counter and sugary drinks in the refrigerator —you are more likely to grab these items out of convenience. In contrast, if your environment (kitchen or desk) is stocked with fresh fruits, nuts, and water prominently displayed, those healthier options become the natural choice. The environment you create will become your natural choice.

Redefining the environment that contributed to your illness may feel uncomfortable, as it challenges familiar routines, but it is a necessary step in building new healing habits. Creating a supportive environment means to prioritize restorative practices for the body to provide it with the raw material it needs to rebuild at the cellular level, practices such as adequate sleep, drinking enough water, eating anti-inflammatory and nutritious foods, and reducing stress and toxins that come from environmental pollutants, including processed foods.

To help your body heal, you must re-evaluate—and sometimes completely transform—your surroundings. Healing cannot thrive in a negative or unsupportive environment, and that unsupportive environment is the reality of where you are now. You must create a new environment that promotes healing and allows progress with less resistance and discomfort.

The principles in this book provide clear guidance on building a healing environment through intentional habits. By focusing on this essential concept and surrounding yourself with positive influences, you'll be well on your way to a healthier, more vibrant version of yourself.

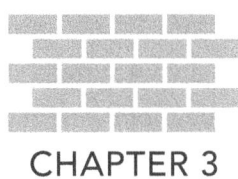

CHAPTER 3

A PRODUCT OF YOUR HABITS

*Life habits do not change until your thinking does.
Shift your mindset, make it your identity,
and everything else will follow.*

You and I are both the product of our personal habits. The habits that rule our daily actions can be our friend or enemy, working either for or against us. In the case of a diseased body, your habits have been working against you, so you need to look at how to make them work *for* you. Managing symptoms and helping your body to heal itself hinges on the fact you make changes to your lifestyle habits.

Habits are behaviors, or actions done automatically and typically without conscious thought. These can be good, bad, or neutral behaviors and as such can be good or bad or neutral for the body. Examples of good habits can be preparing good meals, drinking plenty of water, gratitude, mindfulness, planning and prioritizing your day, or simplifying your life. Bad habits include overworking, lack of physical activity, smoking, and negative self-talk. Neutral habits are actions that don't create a strong emotional reaction or any undue stress on the body such as personal hygiene.

I would like to offer you some grace, as I believe that our auto-pilot, modern lifestyle is full of easy access to bad behaviors and habits that have become root causes of disease. I am convinced that, if asked, you would say that you did not develop these behaviors and habits to consciously poison your system, inflame your gut, or stress yourself out to the point of developing an overrun diseased body. With new awareness, it is your job to identify and replace your harmful behaviors and habits to redefine the environment that contributed to your illness into one that will help your body to heal.

□□□

CHANGING BEHAVIORS

In his book *Atomic Habits* James Clear outlines three layers of how to change your behaviors to change your habits. I will not go into detail here but will paraphrase them to help you understand the challenge of going against the norm to change our lifestyle habits in order to help your body to heal. I have found this to be a good concept to understand when dealing with any change—especially when dealing with chronic illness.

The first layer is trying to change your overall outcome. Outcomes can be described as goals or changes in your overall result, like feeling better.

The second layer is changing your process—your habits and routines—such as developing a new diet, sleep patterns, or reducing stress.

The third layer is changing your identity. This involves looking at your beliefs and self-image along with your judgments and assumptions about yourself and others to see how these affect your choices.

These three layers of behavior changes are principles that allow us to change our lifestyle habits and with specific purpose and correlate directly to reversing our health issues. We can easily understand the goal of helping your body to heal and recognize the importance of identifying specific processes, but many of us overlook the fact that the greatest impact is from changing our identity.

◻◻◻

AN EMPOWERED IDENTITY

I realized after making my decision to manage my disease, it was only just that—a decision—and while an important milestone, it was not getting me to any noticeable improvement in my health or giving me any concrete direction. I was making choices haphazardly and was unsure what improvements I needed or wanted. I hid my illness the best I could by not participating in many of the outside opportunities of everyday life and most importantly I did not really believe deep down that I had even made the 'right' decision—just a stubborn one.

After a very painful flare-up that left me bedridden for days, I realized that something had to change, and it wasn't about my decisions, rest, or diet. I took a deep breath and realized that if I truly wanted to get better, it wasn't about 'wishing' to be better, deciding to eat healthier, or just 'fixing' the flare-ups. It was about changing how I viewed myself and how I viewed my disease. I needed to see myself as the person I wanted to be.

Over the next few months, I worked on making small but meaningful physical changes and adopted a new attitude about healing. I practiced seeing myself as healthy and full of vibrant energy. I took time for myself each day and created routines to calm my anxiety, which I found mirrored my overactive immune system. I detoxed my life, ate clean foods, and set boundaries. Slowly but surely, the flare-ups became less frequent, and my energy returned in a more consistent and sustainable way, which was the beginning of the habits I eventually developed and share with you now. My disease was still present, but I now felt like I had more control, believed I was getting healthier, and saw myself as a healthy person doing things I wanted to do. During my next check-up, the doctor was surprised by my progress. "Whatever you're doing, keep it up."

Those words made me realize that I had changed my identity. *I went from someone who fought against her disease haphazardly to someone who took care to make and embrace the correct choices. By proving to myself that I could heal myself with small wins, I became just what I wanted to be: a person who could manage her disease by listening to her body and who had the power to stop any destructive habits. I was no longer the victim but the empowered healer.*

Your identity defines not only who you are, but who you can become. It is what shapes your thoughts, actions, and purpose. You will never get the wanted results in managing and healing your body if your identity remains that of a victim of a disease or someone who is not or ever will be healthy. Being a victim means you are stuck in feeling that circumstances are beyond your control, hold on to 'why me' thoughts, blame the government or the food manufacturers, or are too reliant on conventional medicine. Change in your identity comes when you move away from thinking like a victim and toward believing in your personal power. A healing mindset is about changing what you identify with.

I found the best way for developing a healing identity is a process of going within, listening to your body, understanding and accepting where you are now, and believing in your intuition. Through this process, you begin to see it is about you finding you in your core ideals and purpose. It is about taking a stand against the establishment, about being your own best friend, health advocate, and superhero. Your identity is knowing who you are and what you stand for.

When any habit becomes part of your identity, it becomes a force that will carry you unconsciously forward, whether it is with an unwanted decline in health or to help your body heal. (Friend or enemy; victim or empowered). The behaviors and thoughts that have currently defined you as a patient diagnosed with a disease and in ill health must be redefined with new behaviors, thoughts, and habits. A goal to help your body heal itself requires a responsibility to oneself to become that person. It is one thing to say, "I am someone who *wants* this," it is very different thing to say, "I am a person who *is* this."

Life habits do not change until your thinking does. Shift your mindset, make it your identity, and everything else will follow.

> **It is one thing to say,**
> **"I am someone who *wants* this,"**
> **it is very different thing to say,**
> **"I am a person who *is* this."**

◻◻◻

MOMENT TO MOMENT: COMPOUNDING SMALL HABITS

There is an operations philosophy utilized in business called Kaizen that focuses on small continuous improvements. I worked for a company that successfully implemented this training and philosophy, and it was interesting to see the immediate results in how the work environment improved productivity while employees became more contented. The basic concept seemed to be counterintuitive when it was first presented, as the first step was not to identify a specific high-level goal but to have a low-level understanding of what frustrated the employees most in their areas and what changes they would make if they could. The second step in the process was to brainstorm ways to make the changes without it negatively affecting colleagues or productivity. Most of the improvements identified and then implemented were very small and were agreed upon by everyone. There were no grandiose remodels or even personnel changes asked for. Instead, it was things like 'store the copy paper close to the copier,' 'answer emails only between 3:00 and 4:00 p.m.,' 'have an on-point fifteen-minute department meeting each morning instead of a weekly two-hour meeting when the issues are old and gone,' or 'being able to collaborate with other departments.'

All were easy changes to implement that made a difference in big ways and were paramount to reaching the high-level management goal. The goal was never really the impetus to drive the changed processes; it was the ability to make small improvements. When we apply this philosophy in our daily lives, we can see that it is easy to underestimate the effect of making continual small improvements that will garner big results.

Where your health is concerned, the small consistent changes which create improvement may seem to have very little impact on your symptoms at first. However, compounded over time, the effects of the small changes become noticeable in a big way. In the example above, not much in terms of productivity would have changed if only the copier paper was relocated, but the compounding of all the small changes and the continual focus on improvement made a noticeable difference. The same holds true that small improvements in our environments and choices each day will go undetected until suddenly one day you realize the debilitating symptoms are no longer present, you feel better, and the disease is in remission. The reverse is also true, in that very little of the destruction happening in our bodies from inflammation or other root causes can be seen or even felt by us until it has compounded to a point you can't ignore. Be assured that things are happening below the surface whether you can see the results or not; for good or ill.

Here is another example of the effect of small decisions. Consider this formula: If you improve just 1 percent each day, the compounding effect results in being nearly thirty-eight times better by the end of a year. Conversely, doing one thing worse each day will take you down to zero. Initially, there is no noticeable difference between the 1 percent better and worse, but over time, the compounding effects become noticeable and definitive (I personally have been there and never want to hit zero again.)

I NEVER WANT TO HIT ZERO AGAIN.

This principle of continual improvement can be applied to your life by adopting and compounding new healthy habits and releasing old unhealthy habits. I have found that everything related to success or failure comes down to the decisions made in the moment. You will have more success setting smaller milestones to work toward than having just an overall goal of 'feeling better.' Lifestyle healing habits are your smaller milestone goals to achieve success. Don't get bogged down by the big picture when it is the moment-by-moment decisions that create small accomplishments that will make a sustainable difference.

In this moment, you may feel you are too sick to ever feel better again, but if you move one step forward, the momentum will begin to carry you toward the health you desire, moment by moment.

□□□

HOW DO YOU MAKE IT STICK?

There are very few of us who have not been introduced to a concept, idea, or improvement plan that we have started excitedly with every intention of success. Then, sometime later, we forget to practice, get to a place of resistance, or become disillusioned by slow results and quit. Despite our efforts and doing all the things, the end result can be a mediocre improvement or none at all. Our good intentions have given way to the path of least resistance, and we remain in our comfort zone. Unfortunately for us now, our comfort zone has made us sick. To move past where we are today and to not only rewire our mindset but create healthy lifestyle habits, we need to train our brain to think differently.

Building a new habit is about training yourself to create a new, consistent response to an event, thought, or action in the moment. An effective way this can be achieved is by attaching the new desired action (the habit we wish to develop) to something you already do. This takes advantage of your natural tendency to go from one familiar action to the next and is an example of "habit stacking," made popular by James Clear in his aforementioned book, *Atomic Habits*. By being consciously aware of what your habits are in a situation and what you wish to accomplish, you will develop sustainable patterns.

For example, say you would like to create a habit of centering your thoughts with a breathing exercise. Each time you sit down at your desk, take three deep breaths and focus on what your current task is. By attaching the breaths to the routine action of sitting down at your desk, you will have more success in the breathing exercise. Another example might be that you want to develop a habit of gratitude each day. If each time you walk into a room you purposefully notice something or someone to appreciate, you will soon make it a habit. The act of noticing your surroundings each time they change will develop that new way of thinking. Attaching new habits to the old familiar behaviors will help improve your success but now let's step it up and do it with intention.

Setting intentions is a common concept, yet an easily overlooked way of creating lasting, desired behaviors. In fact, it is an often-ignored activity in our 'get it done' society. You could say that *without intending to*, you have developed a lifestyle that has led to a chronic illness. Think about what you could do *with intention*.

Intention setting is the practice of clearly defining what you wish to accomplish by focusing on when, where, how, and/or why you carry out a particular action. Look at the previous example of sitting down at your desk and taking three breaths to build the habit of focus and centering your thoughts, and let's add a why. "After I sit down at my desk, I will take three breaths and center my focus to be more productive with my time."

The intention is identified in the why (focus and productivity) and is now attached to the known routine behavior of sitting at your desk. A new habit that can be attached to a routine behavior establishes that mental push but adding the intention will strengthen your commitment. This commitment of the intention is key in making the new habit more automatic and sustainable over time.

CHAPTER 4

HOW TO USE THIS BOOK

When all the pieces are put together, you will realize that you have the power to decide: "How sick do I want to be?"

THE BREAKING POINT

I know it may be exhausting to think about starting anything new—especially when you feel lousy and, as I used to describe it, *"are barely hanging on by your fingertips."* I also know that you will reach a breaking point; a point where you feel you can't take it anymore, a point where you do not want to feel sick, tired, and weak; a point where you want a healthy body more than anything else; a point when you realize the loss of never being able to do that beloved activity again; a point of feeling with a degree of hope that it can all be different and just maybe you can feel well again.

If you are currently at that breaking point, ready to take control, have had enough, are willing to love yourself enough to make a commitment, have decided not to be a victim of your disease anymore, or have just an ounce more energy than yesterday, then *now* is the time to start this journey. By making the decision today to do better by yourself, that last ounce of energy will be well spent.

□ □ □

YOUR FUTURE SELF

Take a moment right now to picture your ideal life in detail, reflecting your deepest desires, hopes, and dreams. See yourself as both the architect drawing the blueprint and the creative visionary breathing life into your dreams with passion. Are you happy, surrounded by loved ones, cheering on your favorite team, climbing mountains, exploring a new travel destination, building a business, doing life with ease and energy?

> **How does it feel to not only survive your days but to thrive in them?**

As your life unfolds in this future vision, believe that each choice you make, each mindful decision, is a building block for a healthier, more vibrant version of yourself. By becoming aware of your thoughts, intentions, and habitual actions, you unlock the power to reshape your reality. This intentional approach allows you to support your body's natural ability to heal and thrive, giving you a greater sense of control over your health and life. Embracing your power to design a life that aligns with your vision, purpose, and the unique beauty of your soul is why you are here.

This book is about the decisions, intentions, environment, and habits I created in my lifestyle that supported my ability to manage symptoms and helped my body to heal itself. This book is about *you* nurturing and caring for *your* body. It is about becoming the best version of yourself and enjoying life to the fullest. If this version of you does not include a chronic illness, then now is the time to make some changes.

The following principles and healing habits are the tools I offer to allow you to manage your symptoms, to identify root causes of your ailment(s), and to help you develop a new lifestyle that embraces the vision you hope for.

As with any work, the more effort and consistency you put into your practice, the more noticeable the improvements will be. I cannot give you absolute or guaranteed results, nor can I say, "Do this three times per day, go here weekly, or eat this and it will all be better."

That type of advice only sets one up for failure. I do not have a magic pill (and no one else does either), but the truth is that, in time, you will hear your own voice of what your body is telling you and that will lead you forward.

I recommend that the principles of "The Decision" and "Your Reason Why" be done first, only because these will help set the stage to show how mindset and identity make a difference in this healing journey. Without making a clear decision and having a clear purpose to be on this journey, it will not be as effective or sustainable. Some of the ideas offered under the healing habits you may be able to implement right away; some take years to come to completion. It has taken years for you to get to this place of dis-ease and there are no overnight quick fixes. Your 'decision' and ' why' will get you through the tougher times.

The Healing Habits sections are the systems and practical suggestions that can be used to develop new habits. The goal is to create the mental shortcuts that create patterns, giving you the ability to take healthy action and make good decisions without conscious thought. You will not need to implement all the habit suggestions, but try as many as resonate in your situation. I encourage you to also come up with a few of your own.

Some Healing Habit sections include a technique you can implement called a "once and done." In these instances, the healthy habit can be accomplished without resistance, thought, or even any continual effort. These are the easy buttons!

As we discussed earlier, illness and root causes are about the whole you, so I have listed some basic emotions related to the topic to develop and those to be aware of. Emotions are a powerful catalyst for transforming your identity to that of an empowered healer. By becoming aware of your feelings in the moment, accepting them, and consciously striving for a more positive emotional state, you open the door to lasting change.

If a principle resonates with you and triggers a physical reaction—like a tightening in your stomach, tears welling up, or a sudden clarity about creating a cleaner environment or maybe addressing a relationship issue, YAY!! That is your intuition speaking and guiding you to the perfect starting point. You will find that your body is going to quickly get on board with your conscious desire to help it to heal itself.

Change is hard for all of us, and you can be assured that taking the *first step* will be the hardest for you, too. It will also be this first step which is the most crucial step *and* the one that promises to make all the difference. The second decision will be easier, and soon you will make good choices and create good habits without even thinking about it. It is all a part of the process, and you will get there. I found it helped immensely to keep a journal or notebook of ahas, problems, lists, things to research, and questions to ask to refer to.

This book offers a fresh perspective, inviting you to explore what might be contributing to your illness, why the disease is a blessing in disguise, and how you can reclaim control of your health—and why it's worth doing so. Through my personal story, I provide an alternative view that goes beyond simply following a traditional medical protocol. I urge you to be willing to look at disease and healing in a different way.

There is an empowering and much more enjoyable option to living life with health management (not disease management) as your goal. Embody the belief that chronic illnesses are much better managed by lifestyle, and you are the architect, visionary, and manager of your lifestyle. Use the experiences, tools, and suggestions here to define what and how that management looks to you.

You are not destined to suffer in pain or become a lifetime victim of your diagnosis.

□□□

The reality is that the lifestyle you have led, the emotions you have held, and the beliefs that you have lived by have, in fact, gotten you to this place of dis-ease. The promise is that today is the first day of the life you want!

Principles and Habits

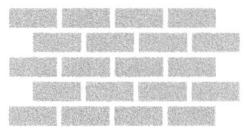

PRINCIPLE 1

The Decision—
This Is Your Game Now

*It is in your moments of clarity that
pivotable decisions are made.*

When I came home from that first hospital visit in 1990, I told my husband the 'angel doctor' had recommended that we go to counseling to help navigate my chronic disease. His surprising response was that this was my problem, not his, and I needed to deal with it. Wait ... what?

His stance (even though made in a loving way) made me just mad enough to stubbornly resolve to take care of myself if no one else was going to do it. Well, wasn't that a revelation?! It was the best thing he could have done for me at that moment.

I felt the victim of my circumstance and old programming surfaced, which fed my initial response to rely on someone to fix me. I didn't like feeling the victim any more than the stubborn anger. Even though it took time to change those mindsets, I realized over time that I really was the only one who could help my body heal itself. I found it was hard at first to look at myself and take responsibility, and I needed to practice making decisions for me. I had not consciously done anything wrong, was living how I had always lived, believed what I had always known and what was 'normal.' But normal wasn't good enough anymore.

I felt blessed that if I had to have a disease, it was one considered to be manageable. And if this could be managed, then I was going to manage it. As those fateful shifts took hold, my mission took shape, and I began studying what might be causing my symptoms, how and why my body was reacting, and then identified how I could change those. Life does not stand still, and each day we are pushed to become the future selves we didn't know we could become.

□□□

TRUST YOURSELF TO TAKE CARE OF YOU

A decision comes with responsibility. Are you willing to take responsibility for the dis-ease in your body? Are you ready to trust yourself enough to take care of yourself? If you are truly serious about making lasting change; if you believe that Western medicine has fallen short of not only managing your disease but helping you reverse this condition; if you have an ounce of belief in yourself, then today is the day to start trusting in you.

Putting trust in yourself is a giant leap of faith in our modern world. Less than 10 percent of humans will consciously take a step forward to depend on themselves, whether it be in business, relationships, or health. If one of your burning desires is to 'help your body to heal itself' then be one of those 10 percent—be the one who goes *all in*.

Think about how we live in a society that teaches us to depend on others for our well-being and works tirelessly to convince us to believe that someone else knows best. We have been taught all our lives to take others' direction and advice, and rarely are we allowed the freedom to listen to and act on our inner knowledge without recrimination—especially in the medical arena. Often, before we have even digested being diagnosed with a disease, we are sent down an unforgiving path of protocol including tests, medications, and surgeries; all the while ignoring that small voice inside that warns that these options may not be the best for us. Others may know scientifically more about your disease, but it is in listening to your intuition of what your body needs that can promote healing and should be honored. *Only* you can do that.

We all have an inner intelligence and intuition that serves us well, and it is wise to develop the art of listening to it and to *trust* in ourselves. You have the power to learn what you need to know, change your habits, and help your body to heal itself. I want to very clearly give you permission to speak up and *trust in you*!

Truth be told, it came as no big surprise to me that when I decided to take responsibility to change my poor lifestyle habits, trust, and take care of myself (with helping my body as the objective), it changed not only my symptoms but my confidence and enthusiasm. I was no longer a victim but empowered. I could see the new me as the *real* me, living as my authentic self. My trust became a decision to be all that I could be, and for me that started with no longer suffering from symptoms of any disease.

Making the decision to take control of your health is a huge leap of faith. Insecurity can be a constant companion, so you need to **stay strong** and **decide** that you will do whatever it takes to help yourself and live the life you want. Use all means necessary within conventional medicine, holistic lifestyle habits, self-development courses, alternative therapies, and even Google searches to achieve your goal.

This decision to help yourself and take control of your own wellness path is not meant to put yourself on an island, just the opposite is true. We want to make ourselves an ally and colleague with our medical team in conjunction with taking an active 'leadership' role in managing our symptoms and illness. As I said, with a decision comes responsibility, and it is now time to step up into that role.

**It is your body, your life, and your disease to deal with.
No one knows better what is best for you than you.
If you continue to do what you've always done,
You will have what you have always had.**

□ □ □

HEALING HABIT 1: THIS IS YOUR GAME NOW

Emotions to develop: Inner strength, Determination
Emotions to be aware of: Imposter Syndrome, Victimization

Your healing starts with permission to become someone different—to create a new identity. Start with where you are today but *decide* who you want to be. Be open to change and break away from the crowd and the status quo. Realize that it may take undoing everything you have known, believed in, and been taught up to now. Take on that executive management role in your life and your health. This is your game now.

- Make a conscious, *out loud decision* that you are going to *take care of yourself* by helping your body to heal itself and do what it takes to make that sustainable. *Declare your decision* and *accept responsibility* that while you may take advice from professionals, family, and other patients, you will *only do what is right for you.*
- Put the statement in writing either in this book, in a journal, on a poster, or as your screen saver to remind yourself.
- Look at your lifestyle with honesty, humility, and with determination decide what *is* working and what *is not* working for you. Decide that you *will* change those things that are

not working. You do not need to know how you will do that today but set the intention.

- Give some thought as to what it means for you to be open to change and accept that there are limiting beliefs you will need to overcome that will try to hold you back. Knowledge leads to power and confidence, so go on a personal mission of self-development to learn whatever you feel unsure of and gain the inner wisdom you need to take care of yourself responsibly.
- Believe this healing journey is possible and that *you can* make a difference in your own health by holding yourself accountable. The following principles will help with that accountability.
- See and begin to love the real you and decide today to support the wins, losses, and challenges that occur during this process. Practice looking at yourself in the mirror and say "hi." Follow the "hi!" with a "good job." "I love you." "be happy!," "we got this," "we can do better." or any other affirmation you feel supports you. This is about you and living your best life. Talk to your body and your body will talk to you, telling you what it does or does not need. Your symptoms are its direct communication.
- Find a quote that supports your courage, your decision, and your desire to heal.
- Work through the following principles of this book with determination. These are your tools to get you away from the pain of where you are now to a place of helping your body to heal itself.

Take back your life and your body. The truth is that no matter where you are today, it is never too late to make the decision, take responsibility, and create new healing habits.

When I made the commitment to help myself, I trusted in myself and believed in myself first and foremost. I was no more special than you and had little confidence in the beginning, but I did have the will to succeed. I was not satisfied with just managing the symptoms, I wanted lasting relief and I wanted my health back. I worked hard at *not* being a victim of my circumstances; changed my identity to one of a healthy, vibrant person; and moved forward to define a life I wanted. If I can do it, you can too. Make that binding contract with yourself.

THIS IS YOUR GAME NOW
A CONTRACT WITH MYSELF

Make the decision official and write a non-negotiable contract to take care of YOU, put yourself and your health first, and do what it takes to make healthy lifestyle choices and develop good habits. Promise neither to give up or to beat yourself up if you backslide a few steps and instead strive to make small improvements each day.

Today, I make the decision to commit to taking care of myself. I promise to honor my body, mind, and spirit, and make healthy choices, with the goal of managing my diagnosis and its symptoms to create my best life. I will do this by:

_____

_____

_____

_____

_____

_____

Signed_____

Dated_____

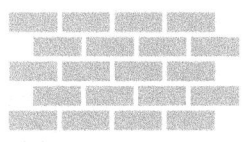

PRINCIPLE 2
YOUR REASON WHY

He who has a why to live can bear almost any how.

−FRIEDRICH NIETZSCHE

I did not want to live in a diseased body. I didn't feel good, had little to no extra energy to spare, and I did not want to live that way. I did not want to take nasty medical tests or medications that gave me worse side effects than the symptoms. I did not want to feel the constant pain. I did not want the uncertainty of what tomorrow would bring. One afternoon, I was complaining, hating, and overall lashing out in a rampage . . . something I tended to do too often. "D*mn the disease, d*mn the doctors, the schedules, the pain, the frustration. I am finished with it all!" I lamented.

When I calmed down, my little five-year-old daughter innocently asked me if I wanted or needed anything. It was a breaking point. I was complaining about a life where my focus was on what I did not want. I realized in that moment it could instead be about what I did want.

I had yet to decide what I wanted. I needed a purpose, a reason to put in the effort, and when I gave it some thought, I found I did have a game-changing reason to want to be healthy. This reason—my WHY—became my driving force to do what it took to heal my body, have energy and vitality, and live what I defined as my new normal life from that day forward.

In my case, I wanted the ability to raise my children as normally as possible. I wanted no restrictions to participate because I was too weak; I wanted to interact, be a part of their lives, and do it without feeling ill. I wanted to feel good, to manage my symptoms better, and to know I was in control of my body. I made this my purpose and my why. I never looked back.

We all have hopes, dreams, and bucket lists—things we want to do with our lives—and this comes with a picture in our head of what our days will look like. When suddenly diagnosed with a disease that may forever change that picture, the shock and sadness invoked can completely derail a person. You may suddenly feel like you no longer have the option to have dreams, and that you will no longer be able to make decisions about your life.

The emotional turmoil is very much a grieving process, and justifiably so. You have been thrown off your path and now find yourself on a very different road, left wondering what life can hold for you now. The life you had pictured or have been working for suddenly grinds to a halt, being replaced with endless doctor and hospital visits, isolation, pain, and anger. It is an emotionally charged situation, and how you handle it can make all the difference.

Many of those diagnosed with an illness are just fine where they are at. They have accepted their disease, declining health, and limitations. They may only feel comfortable following what the doctor prescribes. But if you have found this book, I am betting that you want a little more control of your situation and want a different outcome and path than most. After making the decision to help your body to heal, the very next thought to address is: *what do I want and why do I want it?*

DECIDING WHAT AND WHY

Being derailed by a diagnosis is a shock. It is also a blessing and can be used as a reset to what was not working in your lifestyle. Use this as a defining moment to truly decide what it is you want. Our society raises children to hide their wants and creativity and 'do what is expected.' You may be living with programming from your childhood, enforcing limiting beliefs such as 'you can't be this,' or 'will never be that,' or 'others know best.' I was a product of that mindset. I was programmed to follow what was considered 'normal,' do as expected, and believed that I was not allowed to think outside the box. For you, this may look like anything from not enjoying the job you have found yourself in, to eating fast foods that are the modern social norm, to not allowing yourself to think outside the conventional medicine box. There are enormous amounts of restrictions and expectations that put burdens on our lives that many are unaware of.

I believe one of the leading causes of disease is not being your authentic self or true to what you want and instead living someone else's idea of what your life should look like. When my daughter asked what I wanted, I found that I did not have a good answer, or even a starting point, to determine what I wanted, who I was, or why I wanted it. I was only focusing on what I did not want . . . and I realized that was the mistake.

> **You need to know where you are to get to where you want to be! And you need to know why you want to be there!**

It is important to identify not only your desires but your reason for wanting them. Your intentional decision to put in the effort to help your body heal itself is a good start, but knowing your 'why' will hold you accountable. Just like mine, your reason why will become the driving force to implement and stick to the improved lifestyle habits over the next several weeks, months, and years. It will become the thing that reminds you not to eat donuts just because everyone else is, the reason you are taking walks at lunchtime, and the reason you are putting the effort in each and every day.

Your enthusiasm for life is hidden in what you want and the reason why. Many of us go through life on autopilot, doing what is needed or expected of us in school, jobs, social norms, and caretaking of family. But is that the *real You*? It is important to reconnect with *the you* that wants to come out—*the you* that is defined by your values and ideals.

□□□

WHO YOU ARE AT YOUR CORE

The place to start when determining the real you is to know your core values. These are the things you believe in above all else. No matter how out of control life becomes, you can fall back on these values. When our enthusiasm wanes or our 'why' gets smothered, typically we are doing something that doesn't align with who we are. Knowing your core values helps you to know when and why situations are affecting your health. It is worth the time to stop and identify your core values and where they are not being expressed in your life.

Some examples of core values:

- Authenticity
- Adventure
- Curiosity

- Altruism
- Equality
- Kindness / Compassion
- Creativity
- Nurturing
- Integrity
- Commitment
- Respect
- Courage
- Ambition
- Honesty

Core values are like superpowers, and we all have this superpower within us. An amazing thing will happen once you make the unequivocal decision to live within your core values. You may notice your life unfolding in almost a magical way. Rather than feeling you are swimming against the tide, synchronistic events and coincidences begin to increase, and things go smoother. Suddenly, you find the exact article or meditation you need show up in your social media feed. Or maybe a class at the rec center you have been wanting to take now fits into your time schedule. Or the one food you have not been able to eat suddenly has an organic alternative you can use.

If you were to combine the concept of your **why** (the reason behind your actions) with the **core values** you inherently possess, you would unlock a powerful insight: the discovery of your **purpose**. Your 'why' provides the motivation that drives you, while your core values represent the principles that define who you are. When these two align, you gain clarity about what truly matters to you, leading to a sense of purpose that you can lean on. This is important because living with purpose gives your life direction, helps you make healthy lifestyle choices, and will keep you on track.

> **Discover who you are and why you do what you do, and then do it on purpose.**

□□□

HEALING HABIT 2: WHY + CORE VALUES = PURPOSE

Emotions to develop: Inner strength, Courage
Emotions to be aware of: Discouragement, Anger

I have made thousands of choices regarding my own health over the years, and all were made with my **wants**, **values** and **why** in mind. You also will make thousands of choices throughout your life. Consider your why and core values with each mouthful of food, each decision to rest, each relationship you nourish or run from, each time you choose to *not* let a particular situation get to you. Your *purpose* will keep you on track. I promise that it will make a difference in a big way.

- Identify your core values and write them down to reference when needed. Incorporate what defines you in each area of your life. Defining who you are and what you believe in above all else will help you figure out what types of adjustments you must make to be true to yourself. Begin with answering some straightforward questions:

    Who are you really?

    What is important to you?

    What drives you?

    How do you spend your free time?

    Examine your role models and what you admire about them.

Pay attention to what angers you and what makes you smile.

Where does your integrity lie?

- Identify what is important to you and what makes your life worth living. Make a bucket list as an 'I want list.' Start with a list of twenty-five things you want to *do*, then expand to twenty-five things you want to *have*, and then expand again to twenty-five things you want to *be*. Include things that may seem small, big, seemingly unrealistic, and obtainable. There are no limits here.

- Identify your wants and reasons **why**. The following questions can help you get started on the habit of making, revising, and looking at your why and are an invaluable tool.

    What are your hopes and dreams? What do you love to do?

    Identify the people that are most important to you.

    What is the game-changer in the things you have identified on the previous lists? It needs to be something so important that your life would have no meaning without it.

    What is the reason for the non-negotiable contract you are willing to make with yourself to make the lifestyle changes needed that will help your body to heal itself?

    Why do you want a healthy body?

- Text your *why* to your friends and family, make a poster for the kitchen wall, a sticky note on the bathroom mirror, or make it your screen saver. Look at it every day. Going forward, whenever you feel that you cannot go on, the road is too tough, or the choice is too hard, you will want to remember this reason for working so hard on you:—your *why*. This is a critical step in taking control of your own health. This conviction will become your driving force to go on.

- Visualize the life you want by making a habit of taking a couple of minutes each day to picture that healthy, fun-loving person (you) enjoying life and living your dreams. It is a life that is not restricted by illness, diet, pain, or embarrassing symptoms, but one that is happy, full of vitality, with wonderful relationships and all the success you want. When you can see yourself living the life of your dreams, you begin to change your beliefs. You are telling the universe that "this is how I want to be," and it sets the process in motion. You begin at that moment to heal your body. Make a vision board or write about it in detail.

If you define your purpose by developing your values and knowing your **why,** and dedicate your life to this endeavor, not only will your body respond with joy inside, but the universe will do all that is needed to support you. I am not suggesting that it will be all roses after this declaration, but it will certainly create a brighter path than the one you were on yesterday. Embrace the process and know all is as it should be.

WHY + CORE VALUES = PURPOSE

My Core Values :

My Reason Why:

Gives me Purpose:

PRINCIPLE 3

HARNESSING YOUR FAITH

The wound is the place where the light enters you."

—RUMI

I can remember one day being frustrated by a doctor's visit that did not go well. I was hurting, exhausted physically, and felt beaten down to a pulp, feeling I could no longer handle any of it. I had been reading a book by a Native medicine healer on universal energy and how prayer and drawing down a golden light into the diseased area could help one heal. I had nothing to lose, so I recited the prayer, relaxed, and then pictured myself asking for and receiving a healing golden light to enter my body and surround the affected area. I was amazed that within minutes I felt the physical effect of heat and then calmness in my gut. As I lay there, I also felt an emotional peace I had not been feeling before. As I continued the practice each day or so, I noticed my whole body becoming calmer, and when I tuned into my disease, I began to see it healing. It was like I was suddenly connected to a universal conductor that allowed me to ask for and receive the healing. I continue—an expanded and deepened version of this practice to this day.

Struggles and suffering can lead to healing and transformation, not only in your physical body but in your spiritual and emotional body, as well. Taking responsibility, obtaining the knowledge you need, and then implementing habits to manage your symptoms can look and feel like a big leap off a cliff. It is a leap into the unknown of self-reliance and diligence. It is a leap of faith.

Embracing faith in spirit—whether grounded in a specific religion, a belief in universal energy, or simply in the strength of one's higher self—can be an immensely powerful step on your healing journey. Taking responsibility for your own healing is often overwhelming, especially when it requires you to adopt new habits and let go of old patterns. But this leap of faith—trusting that the process will work, even when it's difficult—is an undeniable act of self-empowerment.

□□□

FAITH IN YOUR BODY

Healing is rarely a straight and easy path. Putting faith in the process means learning to listen to the wisdom of your body, applying practices that require patience, and trusting natural rhythms. Faith is the cornerstone of the listening ability you will need to develop. It creates a connection and a relationship with your authentic self. It is this relationship that becomes a mystical power, giving you sovereignty and control over your own body and thoughts. A habit of tuning in to what your body is telling you—what is causing its dis-ease and how to fix it—is essential. It will create focus, determination, and sustainability in your actions and everyday choices. When you don't stop to think and listen, your actions become quite haphazard—and lead you to the place of illness you are now.

Listening to your body takes some practice but can more easily be accomplished by listening with gratitude, love, an openness, and willingness to help. Your body comes on board very quickly to tell you through intuitive thoughts or symptoms what is going on and how the food, emotion, or stress is affecting it. That distaste for sushi or that pain in your chest during an argument is usually not just coincidence.

Self-development also plays a vital role here. As we strengthen our ability to listen to our inner voice and develop habits that support well-being, we learn to trust ourselves, building the foundation for self-respect and inner peace. This personal trust complements our faith in a higher power, creating a holistic approach to healing that taps into both inner and outer sources of strength.

□□□

FINDING STRENGTH

Faith can function as your anchor on this journey, grounding you in the belief that you are not alone. When you cultivate trust in something beyond yourself—be it a higher power, the interconnected energy of the universe, or the resilience within—you are supported by a vast amount of strength. This higher strength can provide the courage needed to face and work through the obstacles on the path to creating your healing habits. Simply stated, this is not a journey to take alone.

The human condition of pain is a holy place in our bodies. It reminds us of our vulnerability and forces us into a space of humbleness. The pain of an illness, whether emotional or physical, can very often be the catalyst that brings us to our knees and opens us to a place of trust. Trust in our higher self can offer a sense of surrender, which can be a source of relief and freedom from the responsibility of caring for yourself. This surrender is different from the societal norm of feeling a victim of your illness. When you believe that a higher force guides you or that there is a doable path forward, it becomes easier to make peace with where you are in the process. In this way, faith and trust transform the journey of healing into a process of self-discovery and inner growth and force you into the present. This trust must come from belief in yourself.

Many decisions are made without thought, intention, or premise in our daily lives. Faith, trust, and belief are needed to stay in the present moment—the now—to make thoughtful and impactful decisions that will support the healing process. Being present in the moment becomes a grounding habit that allows time for you to stop and think before you act, allows you to be intentional with prayer or meditation, or supports you in that surrender and offers strength that will have far-reaching effects in this journey.

> *"Faith is the strength by which a shattered world shall emerge into the light."*
>
> –HELEN KELLER

□ □ □

HEALING HABIT 3: TUNE IN AND THEN LISTEN

Emotions to develop: Trust, Patience, Humility
Emotions to be aware of: Distrust, Fear, Hopelessness

Powerful spirituality habits that can help you develop a deeper sense of connection, resilience, and inner peace will further your resolve and healing outcome. You want to create habits that force you to tune in and be present to make those good decisions. You may already have some good habits around your faith, and I encourage you to use and develop those fully. I would also suggest that you consider adding a new way to express your faith to expand and grow your own self-development.

- Meditation calms the mind, grounding you in the present, and encourages self-awareness. Practices such as mindfulness, breath-focused meditation, or guided visualizations can help you connect with a sense of inner stillness and deepen your spiritual connection.
- Prayer is about asking for guidance and help. You can ask your body in prayer what it is trying to tell you by simply stating: "Help me. Help me understand what you are trying to tell me." Listen quietly for the answer.
- Intention setting aligns your thoughts with your healing goals. Simply speak or write specific intentions around relief from pain, healing, or clarity. Regularly setting intentions can help focus your mind and open you to higher spiritual insights and your own inner guidance. Practice having faith that with these intentions at the forefront in your mind, your body will respond with answers.
- Deep breathing exercises help you center yourself and connect with your inner energy. Practicing this regularly not only reduces stress but also enhances awareness of your body and soul, grounding you in the present moment.
- Research or take some classes on spiritual traditions and healing practices. The list is endless, but Ayurveda, traditional Chinese medicine, Reiki, shamanism, earth and crystal healing, homeopathy, or sound healing are some to consider. Find what most resonates with you and tap into the interconnectedness these practices can provide.

- Connecting with nature has an innate ability to nourish the spirit and recalibrate the body. Whether it's a walk in the woods, a visit to the beach, or simply watching a sunset, spending time in nature connects you to the natural world and fosters a sense of peace and oneness. It can restore your faith in yourself by showing you the wisdom of the world we live in.
- Engaging in creative activities—like drawing, dancing, or music—can be a form of spiritual expression. Creativity connects you to the essence of who you are, giving voice to feelings and insights that may not emerge through words alone.

Incorporating spiritual practices and faith into your life can build a strong foundation of personal awareness, resilience, courage, and inner peace. It will give you something to hold on to on those days when you are feeling discouraged and less than successful.

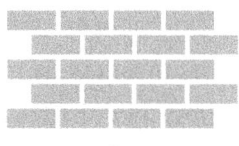

PRINCIPLE 4

THE HAWK'S EYE PERSPECTIVE

"It's not what you look at that matters, it's what you see."

–HENRY DAVID THOREAU, *WALDEN 1854*

I mentioned that when I began writing about my health journey, several symptoms that I had not experienced in several years appeared seemingly overnight. As I worked through the emotional trauma of the diagnosis and what that had meant in my life, I realized there were still current issues that needed to be addressed. During this same timeframe, I was also defining a new relationship, experiencing being a grandmother (including how not to step on the momma and daddy's toes), physically moved to a new city, and started a new job. A whirlwind could describe my life at the time. I realized that even though my healthy lifestyle habits were generally working, and I had been managing my disease well enough, if I was going to keep up the pace, a new plan was in order. Life was growing and changing; I had different challenges and was outside of my normal comfort zone. I wasn't about to let it all make me sick again.

◻◻◻

Perspective is the lens through which we view our lives and how we see and interpret our experiences and navigate the challenges. Just like a hawk that sees the meadow from high in the sky and can zoom in on the slightest movement below, looking at your life with that keen sight will allow you to identify where you are right now. It helps you to recognize patterns; understand connections between symptoms, actions, and emotions; and even identify what truly matters. Without perspective, we risk getting lost in the details—reacting to life's moments without seeing how they fit into our bigger picture. Making a habit of looking at your life with a high-level perspective empowers you to approach your decisions with clarity and purpose and makes room for your intentional healing.

Life is a collection of scattered pieces mixed with responsibility, long-term goals, details of to-do lists, and emotional highs and lows—not to mention illness, symptoms, and fatigue. Taking the time to see the 'big picture' allows you to step back and see how these pieces fit together and to then focus on areas that are going well or need to be rebalanced or done away with altogether. Stepping back gives you clarity on what energizes and depletes you. It helps you identify where you are putting your energy and whether it aligns with your core values and long-term goals. It's about asking yourself, *Does this add meaning or joy to my life?* Without this view, it's easy to fall into routines or habits that might not support your health—which is no doubt where you are now. This awareness can be the catalyst for powerful, healing change.

◻◻◻

EMOTIONAL GUIDANCE SYSTEM

Your emotions are powerful indicators of your current state of health. They provide insight into what you might be ignoring, suppressing, or overlooking. Positive emotions can guide you toward activities and habits that bring fulfillment and joy, while the more negative emotions—like stress, sadness, or frustration—can highlight areas that need healing or adjustment. When you allow yourself to fully experience and reflect on your emotions, you gain a clearer understanding of who you are at this moment and can identify what is serving you and what is affecting your well-being.

Understanding and addressing your emotions and their effect on your symptoms is not a process that happens overnight, and these realizations often come in layers. It requires patience, self-compassion, and a commitment to ongoing self-discovery and perspective. Emotions, especially those deep-seated negative ones tied to past experiences, can take weeks, months, or even years to fully understand and release. This principle is less about rushing to a solution and more about creating space to observe what is going on in your body. You may uncover hidden feelings like anger, guilt, or fear, or you may recognize traits like kindness, resilience, or courage.

Seeing your hawk's eye view is more than just taking a moment to reflect, it is about fully embracing the journey of your life, with all its twists, turns, and pauses. When you see the big picture, you see the connection between where you've been, where you are now, and where you want to go. By tuning into your emotions and recognizing their important role as indicators to symptoms of illness, you can navigate with greater clarity and purpose. This perspective not only empowers you to make healthier choices but also reminds you that developing healing habits is a continuous, intentional process.

> **When you see the big picture, you see the connection between where you've been, where you are now, and where you want to go.**

HEALING HABIT 4: TAKE OFF THE ROSE-COLORED GLASSES

Emotions to develop: Openness, Positive Expectation
Emotions to be aware of: Victimhood, Worry, Blame

It is time to look at your life with a hawk eye perspective by taking in the high-level view and then zooming in, and then being willing to admit to yourself where it all went wrong or where you have it right. Approach this introspection with honesty and without judgment, allowing yourself to explore both the positive and negative aspects in every area of your life, using your emotions as your guidance. Feel where these emotions are in your body by taking a full body assessment, asking, and listening to the symptoms.

Specific areas to address are career, family, relationships, acts of service, unrealized dreams, diet, exercise, spiritual practices, and financial security. The tendency will be to immediately go to the areas and aspects of your life that cause the most angst and stress, but it is critical to note the circumstances in your life that have gone or are going well also.

The following questions can help you get started, but the work is to identify where you are physically and emotionally and how those aspects of you interconnect. There are no wrong or right answers—only the truth of the matter and the facts of the situation. You may find that for each circumstance, it is difficult to acknowledge, a little uncomfortable, or no issue at all. The idea is to gain perspective.

- Some questions to clarify your thoughts in each situation may be:
    Am I good with this?

Ignoring the situation?
Waiting until things get better?
Hating the circumstance?
Feeling there is no control?
Dreaming but not acting on it?
Too exhausted to care?

For example, if you find you are not okay with your income level, you might ask: *Am I good with this?* or *feel there is no control?*

- Journal your thoughts and emotions around these or any of your own circumstances:

    Are you acting lazy about implementing a healthier diet or exercise routine?
    Do you eat too many sweets?
    Are you interested in feeling better physically?
    Are you depressed or feel like no one cares?
    Are you disappointed with the way things have turned out in your career?
    Have you settled for something less than you desire and deserve?
    Are you living in a home that suits you, or are the apartment neighbors driving you nuts?
    Do the important people in your life support or demean you?
    Do you wish you could work full time rather than be a stay-at-home mom?
    Do you want to be a stay-at-home mom or dad?
    Are you being authentic in your values and goals?
    Do you have the freedom to earn, spend, and save money?
    Do you find yourself constantly apologizing to others?
    Are you successful but unfulfilled in your career?

Are there things that need to be said to your spouse, your mom, or your boss to clear the air?

Do you get the rest you feel you need, or are you 'doing' to the point of exhaustion?

Do you overschedule yourself? Why or why not?

Are your children overscheduled?

Do you feel that you neglect your children?

Are you feeling guilty eating foods you know aren't healthy because it is easier?

Is your spiritual faith in a higher power solid? Missing? Nurtured?

Do you feel insecure in yourself?

Do you wish you had more time to be creative in a hobby you like?

Do you feel guilty that you do not know how to cook? Keep house? Make more money?

Do you trust your doctor but feel resentful that he should be doing more for you?

Are you angry at your body and limitations?

- As you create your list of what your life looks like today, awareness can release some internalized (buried) emotions, and you may find yourself angry, hurt, or frustrated. You may start to experience pain or other symptoms. Don't let that stop you! Awareness is key to releasing and the opportunity to help your body heal itself.
- Stop and do the following in gratitude:
    1. Realize that you cannot change what you are not aware of.
    2. Bless the symptoms and their related emotions and realize the strength in that awareness and ability to move forward.

3. Recognize that your emotions are a direct result of your reaction to the situation. This reaction will give you amazing insight as to the root cause of symptoms.

- Create a seperate list of at least twenty-five things that you love in your life that make you smile. Take stock and brainstorm all the good things, accomplishments, wins, loving friends, and family you have. In what ways are you most proud of yourself? What do you most enjoy? Notice how you feel when you think about these things and note your attitude, emotions, and physical symptoms. You may even place a happy face next to the things you love most!

□□□

**What puts a smile on your face?
You need a lot more of that.
What makes you 'spitting' mad?
You need a lot less of that.**

GOOD THINGS IN MY LIFE

Recognizing accomplishments, loving friends, beauty, all the things that make me Smile.

-
-
-
-
-
-
-

BAD THINGS IN MY LIFE

Recognizing stresses, disappointments, all the things that make me sad and angry and in dis-ease. (Use additional pages as needed.)

-
-
-
-
-
-

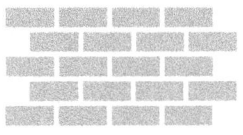

PRINCIPLE 5
TURN 180 DEGREES

> Emotion is the silent architect of our being, whether building resilience or laying the groundwork for illness

It was a struggle in the beginning to decipher what might be causing my symptoms. I was so busy with the everyday needs and challenges of my life that stopping to think about myself did not seem to be worth the time it took. But, over time, with a desire to feel better, I began to look at my life as a collection of circumstances which allowed me to see a clearer picture. By seeing life cut up into blocks of time, I could typically, without fail, pinpoint the things I was doing or the emotions I was feeling that were the cause of my symptoms, and with that knowledge was able to well, honestly, stop doing them. Sometimes it was what I was eating or the stress of overworking, while at other times it was worrying over significant life changes like a daughter leaving for college or starting that new job. Some symptoms hit immediately (e.g., milk products causing diarrhea, or being in the hot sun too long causing weakness), then there were many more that tended to be a slow build. In my case, often it was the smaller overlooked patterns that I just dealt with that built into bigger problems, like not getting outside enough or expectations that didn't sit well with me. Being able to see my life from a higher perspective, I was able to zoom in on each specific problem area.

Sometimes, the best way forward is to turn around. By looking with our hawk's eye view, we can see where life often requires a 180-degree shift—a complete change in direction. This doesn't mean failure or starting over; it means recognizing when the current path isn't aligned with your true needs or authentic self. Turning around is an act of courage and clarity, driven by your ability to see the bigger picture and listen to the signals your symptoms are sending. By shifting your perspective and embracing a new course, you create space for healing, growth, and a life that feels more authentically yours.

In the previous principle, you took a hard look at your life, the things that made you smile, the things that made you spitting mad, and the things you could do more and less of. It is now time to make changes and develop new habits that promote a healthy body. This is where the 'rubber meets the road.' The next step down our path of self-care is to identify where we need to turn—maybe fifteen, ninety, or 180 degrees. Now is the time to make the decision and redefine the areas of your life that aren't serving you; those that drain your energy, create stress, or clash with your core values. (i.e., the areas that literally make you sick). You also need to commit to more of the things that make you smile.

What you choose to spend your time doing and how you react to the life you have created is of utmost importance. Are you going to settle for or justify the painful, bumpy, unhappy road you are on *or* see your current lifestyle for what it really is (a symptom maker) and *change course now?*

◻◻◻

THE COURAGE TO CHANGE

Sometimes we just need to be reminded that our life is our own to create. It is yours and yours alone (no ifs, ands, or buts), determined by your choices and actions. I do not believe that any of us are destined to suffer if we choose not to. You do not have to live a life that is not truly aligned with your authentic self. Take care of yourself and change what needs to change; believe that it is possible, and believe there are no limitations.

One of my favorite quotes is from a movie called *We Bought a Zoo*, and while I don't remember it exactly, it goes something like this:

"Sometimes all you need is twenty seconds of insane courage; twenty seconds of just embarrassing bravery. I promise you, something great will come of it."

Change often feels daunting, requiring a level of courage that seems out of reach. This quote reminds us that transformation doesn't demand constant bravery; it asks for brief, decisive moments of courage. These small, courageous acts can break the cycle of blame, victimization, and depression that keeps us stuck in unhealthy situations. While it's natural to fear the unknown, embracing those small moments of courage can move us forward in powerful ways.

I want you to know you are not alone if change is hard or fearful for you. Even though you may know situations are wrong in your life and recognize their contribution to your illness, it is easier many times to not rock the boat and stay in that comfort zone you are accustomed to. The key to success here is two-fold:

1. Break down the big process into moment-by-moment decisions, focusing on small improvements.

2. Believe in yourself, that it is not too late, and it is something you are capable of. Belief is an attitude that starts with saying, "I can do this."

Sometimes, change can be easier by focusing on and choosing those things that make you smile. It is much easier to make changes when it is an activity or desire that makes you happy.

> *"To be a star, you must shine your own light, follow your path, and don't worry about the darkness, for that is when the stars shine brightest. Always do what you are afraid to do."*
>
> —RALPH WALDO EMERSON, AUTHOR

□ □ □

HEALING HABIT 5: THE COURAGE TO TURN AROUND

Emotions to develop: Confidence, Optimism
Emotions to be aware of: Blame, Boredom

It is time to pull out the decision you made to help your body heal and take responsibility for doing what it takes to put that into practice. In the healing habit of removing the rose-colored glasses, you identified the areas of your life that need to change as you looked at bad physical habits and those that created emotional upheaval. While it may not be easy to find a new job, pack up the house for a move, confront relatives, or distribute new chores to family members, the effort is temporary and very doable. It may take getting rid of the situation or finding the strength to resolve and overcome it. Take the first step with courage. I promise something great will come of it. As you commit to turning the current habit or belief 180 degrees, keep the following principles in mind.

Think of your purpose and reason why
Be grateful for the clarity these situations have given you

Detoxing your life is a must to get the upper hand to manage illness and promote healing

Courage and security come with positive action

- Using the lists already created in the principles of "The Hawk's Eye Perspective" and "Take Off the Rose-Colored Glasses," work with the issues that you **may not be pleased with** (or which you see are creating negative emotions). Begin identifying and creating new habits that work towards accomplishing the turns and changes needed. Start with a root cause and then what the possible solution may be.

  For example, one of the issues you may have identified could be, "I feel guilty eating foods I know aren't healthy." Your answer may be: "Yes, I do need to stop this habit of eating whatever I can grab quickly, I do feel guilty but also justified because I am busy. The way I will turn this around is to pre-plan my meals and purchase healthier snacks to grab and go." In this scenario, being busy is the cause, and pre-planning is the new habit to develop.

  Or, for instance, you may feel like you are trapped in your career. "I am going nowhere fast at this company and am beginning to hate going to work." Your ninety-degree turn may look like, "Knowing how much stress and resentment working at this company is causing, I will first ask for a raise or promotion that will make me feel more appreciated." Or a 180-degree turn could be making the decision to begin looking for another job. Seeing resentment as an emotional energy drain and symptom maker, brainstorm ways to put yourself in a happier position.

- An emotional area identified may be dealing with roles in

your primary relationship. You may see this as no big deal, as you grew up with defined male and female roles in the home, but deep down it irritates you that your partner never picks up their own dirty clothes. A 180-degree turn might look like, "I will ask for help and let my feelings be known that I feel like a doormat."

By identifying the irritation and belief it arises from, you can develop the habit of expressing your emotions in a way that supports you.

- Some ideas to think about that could help you with these changes could be:

    Do you need help or support?

    Do you need a new job or just a heart-to-heart talk with the boss?

    Do you need to set some boundaries with someone in your life?

    Can you establish a monthly girls' night out?

    Maybe a fresh look of new paint and curtains for the dining room will raise your mood.

    Getting more rest this week or just saying no to the latest non-essential request. This may be a quick and easy solution.

    Is it time to be creative and unpack your paints and canvases again or time to dust the piano off?

    Some things may take some time, such as going back to school to have that career you want. Start with a plan of action.

    Sometimes it does not take a physical change at all but a

- change in your emotional reaction to a situation. Attitude is everything.

- Next, for each item on your ***love and makes you smile list*** of good things, decide how to work it into your life as often as possible. If it is a relationship, then nurture it by whatever means necessary. If it is training for a marathon, then run as much as you are able to without putting stress on your body. Celebrating the good things over and over allows you to easily create the attitudes of gratefulness and happiness that will help you heal.

Everyone makes difficult decisions and is navigating challenges in their lives—whether dealing with an illness or not. The key is to allow yourself the grace to work through it at your own pace, but don't let yourself off the hook. Big changes start with a desire to have something different and the courage to start small.

THE COURAGE TO TURN AROUND
TURN 180 DEGREES

What puts a SMILE on your face? You need ALOT more of that. What Makes you Spitting MAD? You need a lot LESS of that.

Hint: I can say no to my friends sometimes to change feeling pressured.

I can do this .... to change this...........................
I can do this .... to change this...........................
I can do this .... to change this...........................

**I get ANGRY... I get HURTFUL...I get STRESSED
I am CALM... I am NURTURING...I am HEATHLY**

Practice turning an unhealthy emotion and action into a healthy one.
- tired & yelling   **can become**   rest and alone time
- angry with food choices   **can become**   thankful of so many healthy options
- ....can become ....
- ....can become ....

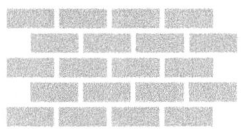

PRINCIPLE 6
STANDARD PROTOCOL

"No man is free who is not master of himself."

–EPICTETUS (DISCOURSES, C. 108 AD)

A year after I was diagnosed with my illness, my daughter was diagnosed with asthma, and three years after that, my husband was diagnosed with Multiple Sclerosis (MS). I had already developed a 'how can I help myself first rather than rely only on conventional medicine?' mindset, but I now wanted to apply that in a caretaker role. When I asked the pediatrician what had caused the asthma, the answer was a list of possible triggers to avoid and reassurance that it was a 'normal' childhood illness. I could understand the triggers, but normal? Not in our world.

After asking the neurologist what could be done to prevent some of the debilitating flare ups my husband was experiencing, we received the medical summation of lifetime medications, infusions, and an eventual wheelchair that they told us would be needed. Just as in my case five years earlier, while I appreciated the medical diagnosis, the prognosis and treatments were frustrating. I didn't want a 'normalized' answer, and when pushed, the neurologist replied with a wavering answer of, "Well, I guess, he could try to not stress the body in any way, shape or form."

In this response, pulled dramatically out of him, I found a nugget of pure gold.

Western conventional medicine is unmatched in its ability to provide fast, life-saving treatments and excels in acute care and emergencies. The scientific research and focus of the how the systems, DNA, and cellular components of the human body all work is nothing short of miraculous. Diagnosing and treating diseases often involves examining how the affected systems of the body are malfunctioning and by using medications, surgery, or other interventions to alleviate symptoms and temporarily slow the progression of the disease, all of which are very much needed. But ongoing management, identifying root causes, and helping the body to heal fall under a different modality of care.

□ □ □

ONLY TREATING THE SYMPTOM

We must realize that conventional medicine has a downside in its quick and immediate emphasis on only treating symptoms rather than addressing underlying causes, particularly for chronic conditions.

The mentality to match a drug with the symptom leads to an emotional over-reliance on medications that never gets to the root of the problem. It's like taking ibuprofen for muscle aches but continuing the activity that caused it. We have been conditioned to believe that this quick fix is enough. Your symptoms will continue to surface and the damage continues to accumulate when you do not eliminate the cause that made your body ill. The pain relief effect of the ibuprofen will eventually wear off, leaving you with sore muscles once again. The solution we are looking for is to help your body heal and to reduce your symptoms. The root causes need to be identified and eliminated as much as possible. Masking the problem is not a solution.

I encourage you to take the medications, do the tests, and follow protocols that have been prescribed until you or your doctor feel you do not need to. Conventional medicine needs to be used congruently with your management of identifying and reducing root causes. Medications are good for feeling some relief, allowing your body to recover from intense symptoms, and helping your mind and emotions to be in a better place. When we partner our healthy lifestyle habits together with conventional treatments in the correct way, progress can be made and success achieved in helping your body to heal itself.

> **The goal is to rely less on conventional medical treatment and more on yourself and your lifestyle to manage your disease.**

As mentioned before, we have become overly dependent on conventional medicine to fix our every ailment. It is in this over-reliance and expectation of drugs being a cure-all that you need to be wary of, believing it to be the only management tool you have. The continual barrage of medications, doctor visits, tests, and prescribed treatments creates a reliance on conventional medicine that fuels your identity of being an ill person and a victim.

Changing your identity to someone helping your body to heal is about changing the thought process. When experiencing chronic or worsening symptoms, you need to make a habit of thinking first, *what is my body trying to tell me?* and then reaching for a lifestyle habit that supports you to eliminate the root cause rather than just turning to the doctor and a medication. Masking symptoms puts undue stress on the body, and when the body is using its energy to recover from stress (in any way, shape, or form), it is not rebuilding healthy cells. It is a fine balance of knowing when medications become the problem not the solution, and my point is to make you aware and question the process. If truth be told, very few of us enjoy being reliant on medications and protocols. It is time to own that truth for yourself.

While you develop new habits to support your body, you will also need to release old habits and beliefs. Reliance on conventional medicine and its quick symptom fixes will be one of those habits. Appreciating where your reliance on conventional medicine is today and developing the habit of taking responsibility for your own health may be the biggest shift you will make in the healing journey. Reflecting on all that you have learned about core values, your 'why,' and the decisions and intentions you now have will help you start to realize what needs to go out of your life. It will be well worth it.

Don't stress the body in any way, shape, or form.

◻◻◻

HEALING HABIT 6: WITH A GRAIN OF SALT

Emotions to develop: Self-reliance
Emotions to be aware of: Doubt, Dependence

Your healing habits are to be used in conjunction with and in addition to your current conventional medical treatments. The goal is to rely less and less on conventional medical treatment and more and more on yourself and your lifestyle to manage your disease; but start where you are right now. Your body is in fact diseased, and you have been diagnosed with a chronic illness. You may currently be taking medications or have had surgeries to help correct or remove damaged areas of the body. Allow this to be your starting point. While standing at the starting block, also be looking toward your destination, be open, and look outside the box to find new ways to support your healing.

In your healing lifestyle, *your* responsibility is to get into the habit of doing the following:

- Develop a habit of thinking first: *what is my body trying to tell me?* Ask yourself: *if I knew the answer to why I am sick and why I have this particular disease, what would it be? Is it an emotional issue? A childhood trauma? A physical toxin or allergy? When did the symptoms begin? What was going on in my life at that time, or maybe several years before, causing stress?*

- Do your due diligence to thoroughly research the specifics of the disease, including its causes, symptoms, and stages. Review various treatment plans, including conventional, alternative, and supportive therapies to understand the range of options and how they might complement each other to work for your benefit.

- Look into each available or prescribed medication, understanding not only why, when, and how it is commonly used but also the potential outcomes, side effects, and the ways it will interact with your body.

- Be willing to stand up for yourself and speak with your medical team about what you are NOT willing to endure for treatment. Many medications and treatment protocols have psychological effects such as personality changes, depression, and anxiety. Conventional long-term disease management tends to work for a time and then not, which can lead you on an emotional roller coaster by being uncomfortable or emotionally draining.

- Decide where your comfort lies in managing your disease—don't blindly accept the decision of your medical provider if that is not what you are inclined to do. Make your own decisions that support your comfort level.
- Take everything you read and the information found on the internet as it applies to your situation with a grain of salt. In other words, due diligence applies to separating what is real and true from the chaff.
- Spend time remembering your beliefs, your purpose, and your desired lifestyle to know what will best suit you. There are no right or wrong answers here, but do not jump on the wrong path just because you were told that is the 'normal' thing or that it may be the easiest or the latest new fix. Understand what the implications both mentally and physically are to YOU if a particular path is chosen.
- Do a deep dive into answering the following questions to help you visualize your identity as it reflects who you are today. Identify the intentions needed to develop your healing habits.

    How has this diagnosis changed your mindset and lifestyle now that you are a potential patient for life?

    What is your identity around your disease today?

    How do you see yourself managing the disease and its symptoms, three months, six months, one year, three years, and five years down the road?

    Is conventional medicine serving you in the ways you want?

How you use conventional medicine is a choice you will need to make for your own situation, but realize that it may be working from a point of disease management rather than health management. Make an informed decision. Know with confidence what you are getting into. Do not settle for additional symptoms or side effects to satisfy what is a conventional or convenient treatment if you do not feel comfortable with that. There is, without fail, a holistic alternative to develop into a habit you can work with. Do not blindly put your healing in another's hands, only to be disappointed and become distrustful, or worse, feeling like a personal failure or victim, if it does not have the desired effect. Be willing to say "*No*—that is not what is right for me, my body or my lifestyle!"

Be STRONG!

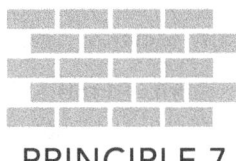

PRINCIPLE 7
DETOX YOUR ENVIRONMENT

To honor the sacredness of our planet, we must commit to detoxifying its lands and waters. To honor the sacredness of our bodies, we must commit to detoxifying its cells.

When my daughter was diagnosed with asthma, it came as another out-of-the-blue inflammatory disease that our seemingly healthy lifestyle did not accommodate. Receiving nothing but an assurance that asthma was not uncommon, a list of possible triggers, and a pack full of inhalers, we were sent on our way. After several years of seeing her suffering severe attacks around Christmastime, we theorized that she was having an allergic reaction to the live Christmas trees we preferred. This seemed quite counterintuitive, as we had mountain property where she could run amongst the trees with no problem. In an aha moment after doing some research, we concluded it was the fire retardant and preservation chemicals sprayed on the lot trees we were buying in town that was the problem. With continued research, it was much easier to keep her away from chemical triggers, reducing the number and severity of attacks throughout the year.

ENVIRONMENTAL POLLUTANTS

It is hard not to listen to any social or news report today that doesn't include evidence of the toxicity of our environment. Our food has long been fertilized and produced with pesticides and chemicals that are toxic to our bodies. Lotions, soaps, and laundry detergents are laden with toxic chemicals that soak in through our skin. People are being diagnosed with food allergies, asthma, and diabetes, and more, all related to what we eat and breathe. We do live in a toxic environment, and the toxins in the body cause diseases—especially chronic illnesses.

The first and foremost way to help your body heal and reduce your symptoms from any chronic illness is to take control of the amount of toxins in your life. Your body is unequivocally telling you it is being poisoned by the many chemicals, plastics, and toxins that enter it.

Realize that as wonderful as your body is, you need to help it in any way you can, and that includes not subjecting it to chemicals it does not know how to deal with. It has been proven that the effect of toxins on our bodies and emotions are such a main root cause of disease that this may well be your most successful principle to employ. While it would be a stretch to believe that you can remove every toxin from your environment, you can consciously reduce them, which will help immeasurably. Reduce exposure by developing habits to eliminate as many substances that can act as poisons as possible.

◻︎◻︎◻︎

EMOTIONAL TOXINS

Many of our normal everyday activities are causing negative, lower vibrational emotions, and it is important to identify these. Stories in the evening news of mass shootings, catastrophic diseases, natural disasters, war, and political issues create a myriad of toxic emotions, including anxiety and anger. Our economy is tenuous at best. Money and family issues can create stress and overwhelm.

Have you ever been in a situation where you have had a reaction of sudden tightness or uneasiness in your stomach? Have you felt sudden nausea when confronted with a situation outside of your comfort level? Do you get a headache each time you talk to a certain person? Have you felt deflated or exhausted after being out with a group you seem to tire of quickly? These are examples of how toxic emotions are directly related to your physical body.

Emotions are created by reactions to a situation. When you react negatively, it lowers your vibrational energy or life force. Traumas, fears, anger, regrets, feeling overwhelmed, and criticism are some of the most common toxic emotions. Awareness is the first step to remedying the cause and allows you to step back and realize that the emotion of the situation needs to be released so that it has no time to cause your body stress. These emotions, if not reduced or let go of properly, stay buried in our bodies and over time are one of the root causes of all diseases. Each time you feel a lower vibration, it affects your healing negatively and has a direct relationship to creating symptoms.

As mentioned before, relationships and people can also be toxic to your lifestyle and emotions. If you have someone in your life who sabotages your attempts at a healthy lifestyle, makes you feel less than you are, or creates pressure to live a way contrary to your values and beliefs, you know how hard that can be on your health. Look inside and trust your instincts about whether you have relationships that are toxic to you. It may take setting boundaries or ending the relationship altogether. You decide.

HEALING HABIT 7: REPEL TOXIC WASTE

Emotions to develop: Positive expectation, Hopefulness
Emotions to be aware of: Frustration, Irritation

Detoxing your environment of chemicals, people, negative emotions, and bad habits will not be accomplished overnight and, in fact, will be a continuous decision. With practice and clarity, it will become easier to make those everyday choices on what you can have in your life to support your good health and what you do not want any part of. The first step is to be willing to make the effort to look at the things you consume and live with a different way and take action to stop putting what is making you sick into your body.

- **Once and done:** Invest in a household water filtration system that suits your home and lifestyle. Beware of plastic toxins from bottled water.
- Go through your food cupboards and take note of how many chemicals or additives there are in the things you put in your body. You can find organic, chemical-free options for anything you use daily. There was a time that the additional cost was significant, but that is not usually the case now.
- Personal care items are also a point of concern. There are so many excellent, organic, sustainable products that you will enjoy much more, knowing they are not poisoning your system. Make it **once and done** by adopting an organic chemical-free brand that you like and make it the only option you buy.
- Get out and enjoy clean fresh air, sun, and nature as often as possible. Being outdoors and in nature promotes good lung, blood, and digestive functions and is an instant stress reducer.

- **Once and done:** Invest in a salt lamp and air purifiers to clean your inside air. Indoor air is full of concentrated pollutants.
- Limit time in front of your electronic devices, including the television, computers, phones, and video games. Radiation and electromagnetic energies wreak havoc in our bodies. Use the speaker on your cell phone whenever possible. Do not charge your devices close to your sleeping area. Invest in EMF devices.
- Medications are toxic to your body. While they may seem to be doing good things, know that they also are creating unseen side effects. To counteract some of the side effects while taking the meds and especially after stopping them, include detoxifying foods such as ginger, green tea, aloe vera, turmeric, and lemon in your diet.
- Look at your relationships with friends, family, and coworkers. How do these relationships hurt or help your healthy lifestyle? Make the decision to let in only those who support your healing wholeheartedly. If that is not an option, then limit their insight into your journey. Put another way—only tell them what you want to. I have found many times that once you are committed to making a healthy habit your norm, others will notice and jump on board.
- Go on a social media hiatus and use the time to research alternative holistic treatments. Watch less news and TV and, don't get emotionally involved in causes and incidents you have no control over. Instead, say a blessing over the situation and release It.

Detoxifying our living environment can be one of the most challenging obstacles to overcome while developing our new habits, but it will yield the greatest rewards. I encourage you to forever make this a part of your daily lifestyle and healing habits for the long run.

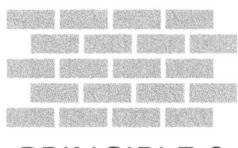

PRINCIPLE 8

DIET AND NUTRITION

"Let food be thy medicine and medicine be thy food."

−HIPPOCRATES

When I began to see that processed foods and lack of nutrition were the culprits of my disease, I initially started slowly replacing the products our family used. This is a perfect case of not waking the sleeping bear of resistance or change too fast for sustainability, as the pushback and tantrums of eating something new were inevitable. As I bought groceries each week, I replaced some of the old standards with healthier or organic brands to make it easier on the whole family to 'digest.' Our refrigerator eventually held more fresh food, and the pantry had more whole ingredients to cook with than prepackaged quick meals. I would encourage the kids to experiment with creating fruit and protein shakes, and supplements of aloe vera and vitamins served us well for many years. When I was diagnosed with cancer, I took a hard look at what had crept back into my pantry and what I was eating on a regular basis. I spent several hours literally filling bag after bag of processed foods, mixes, sauces, and snacks that contained all the wrong ingredients and were filled with toxins that were supporting cancerous cells. After an evaluation and reset, all is once again well.

Your doctor may or may not endorse the fact that diet and/or nutrition plays a major role in disease management. Many doctors still hide from any nutritional and diet advice, but in our world of symptoms, we know that different foods seem to be good for us and others not so much. What I want you to become aware of goes much deeper than whether a certain food is causing immediate symptoms or not.

The principle here is that it is not the kinds of foods or what you eat when or how often. It is the nutrition, or lack of it, and the elimination of poisons (**toxins**) in foods that we need to be aware of for long-term, sustainable healing in our bodies.

Acknowledging a few key concepts in creating our healing and sustainable lifestyle where food is concerned is an important place to begin. I am not a medical professional, nutritionist, or dietitian, but an informed patient who has studied foods and nutrition for over three decades with a personal history and common-sense approach.

- *Foods themselves are not the root cause of the disease.* Your body is reacting to toxic chemical pesticides, fertilizers, processing, and GMOs as dangers. These allergens and toxins in foods send the immune system into overdrive, which is by definition an autoimmune disease and will cause any number of chronic illnesses. Over time, these processed, toxin-ridden foods will cause every person some kind of disease in his or her body. *At the very least, you need to stop bombarding your body with things it is constantly having to fight against, and this means, most importantly, chemically-laden and GMO-processed foods.*
- *Strengthening the immune system* is crucial. Anti-inflammatory foods and natural supplements with immune-boosting properties need to be a staple in your diet.
- *The human body is constantly regenerating new cells.* To heal and sustain good health, it is crucial to supply new cell

development with the most nutritious substances we can. Good, clean foods and water that supply the proper nutrition are the only way to accomplish this.

- *It is your responsibility to be aware of how nutritious your diet is or isn't and adjust accordingly.* At times, it seems the most processed foods cause the least symptoms, but it also goes without saying that these foods also provide no nutrition and are sustaining the disease and its symptoms rather than healing.

THE 'NORMAL' STANDARD AMERICAN DIET (SAD)

It is no coincidence that 90 percent of the foods we eat today did not exist one hundred years ago, and 90 percent of diseases did not exist either. The world of health took a major turn in the 1920s-1930s, when processed oils came onto the scene, and at the same time, many natural remedies were either outlawed or socially denounced. In the 1950s, food 'manufacturers' started to tout convenience above all else. "Work and play—no need to spend hours cultivating and cooking your foods—we can make foods for you!" became a national advertising campaign that forever changed the face of our diets.

The phrases 'food manufacturers' and 'make foods' should have alerted us.

It is understandable that very few of us eat optimally for healing or sustaining good health. Even if we cook most of our meals ourselves, our 'normal' Standard American Diet (SAD) is full of processed foods with little to no nutritional value. Fast food restaurants to high-priced eateries also fall victim to manufactured or GMO foods. Everything from protein products to vegetable oil is mass-produced in the cheapest way possible, which means much of our food includes synthetic chemical compounds, hormones, pesticides, and any number of things that are toxic to our human bodies. This is not new radical information, but it does take a concerted effort to change the way we think and eat.

Dairy, eggs, and red meat are not bad foods. It's also true that fruits and vegetables are not always good foods. The most important thing to remember is that foods laden with toxins or with *no* nutritional value should not be considered normal or good for you. The body needs a plethora of trace minerals, vitamins, proteins, carbohydrates, fats, and of course water to function optimally. In your research, learn what is best for your particular body type. Many nutritionists and dieticians offer these services. This does not mean forever sacrificing delectable, tasty food or even the foods you enjoy. It does mean eating food for nutrition first and foremost.

Four thoughts related to diet and nutrition that you *must adopt* to support the symptom-free lifestyle and heal your body are:

1. *Get over the idea that you eat only for pleasure or to satisfy your appetite.* Foods need to be consumed to *feed your body*, not to please your taste buds. Your body only focuses on what it can digest, uses it to fuel the muscles and systems, and provides nutrition to the cells—not how good the hamburger or cookie tasted. It must also be understood that while your system is compromised with active disease, any filler foods that you ingest are only putting more stress on the system. The filler foods include non-nutritious, processed, and sugar-laden snacks.

2. *Stop eating any food you know is causing you present problems.* It seems obvious, but we have all been there! If you are running to the bathroom with each bite of ice cream, then respect yourself enough to stop eating ice cream. If red meat is causing muscle or joint pain, stop the red meat for a while. If your system is not healthy enough to assimilate

nutrients from fresh vegetables, then find a different preparation for them. Until your body has less inflammation and can digest and assimilate certain foods again, honor the symptoms and find an alternative way to get that nutrition. Blaming or hating the disease because you can't eat what you want at that moment will not get you to a healing place.

3. *Allow yourself to eat what is best for you without self-incrimination or feeling abnormal.* It is much easier now than it was years ago to say, "I can only eat this or that," as it is more commonly recognized to have special diets.

   Shopping today for natural or organic foods is as easy as shopping for processed foods. Restaurants will accommodate most special requests without fuss, and it is also more and more normal to reach for a healthy snack. Redefine your normal to suit your needs.

4. *Eat whole foods that are primarily organic.* Whole foods are foods that exist in nature, and we eat them as nature intended. Fruits, vegetables, grains, nuts, seeds, and animal products such as beef, fish, poultry, pork, and eggs are all whole foods. Whole foods are much easier on our systems than combined foods. If it has more than one ingredient, it will be harder to digest and may be much less nutritious. Whole, unprocessed, or minimally processed dairy products can also be tolerated without distress more than ultra-pasteurized dairy products.

You need to be aware of how nutritious your diet is or isn't and adjust accordingly. Feeding healthy cells is the goal!

HEALING HABIT 8: EAT TO FEED

Emotions to develop: Enthusiasm, Positive Expectation
Emotions to be aware of: Discouragement, Anger

Diets (as in what we eat) are specific to each of us, and there is no one answer that fits all. Your 'perfect diet' will be a combination that suits **your body and your preferences**. This is not about quantity but quality of eating. The habit to master is how you accomplish healthy cell development by taking control of what you feed your body, making it as nutritious as you can, while causing as few symptoms as possible.

Some ways to accomplish this are:

- Start with an evaluation. Keep a journal of everything you eat and drink during a week's time. Next to each entry, note if it is processed (P), whole (W), fresh (F), or filler (X).
    - *Processed foods* are manufactured, altered, cooked, and packaged through various methods. They include added ingredients like sugar, salt, fats, dyes, and chemical preservatives. These are convenience foods requiring little to no preparation. Examples of processed foods include canned soups, deli meats, packaged snacks, sugary drinks, condiments, frozen meals, and baked goods.
    - *Whole foods* are as close to their natural state as possible without a combination of other foods. Whole foods can be minimally processed but are free from artificial additives, preservatives, and

flavors. Examples of whole foods include fresh fruits, vegetables, whole grains (like brown rice or quinoa), nuts, seeds, and lean proteins.
  - Fresh foods are those that have been recently harvested or prepared and have not undergone any significant processing or preservation methods. Examples of fresh foods include freshly picked fruits and vegetables, freshly baked bread, and fresh cuts of meat or fish.
  - Filler foods and snacks refer to items that provide minimal to no significant nutritional benefits, are primarily a source of empty calories, and simply satisfy hunger without contributing essential nutrients.
- Note how nutritious each food on your list is for your body. (You could use a one- to three-point system.) The purpose is to become aware of what you are actually putting in your mouth and how much nutrition it is or is not providing for you. Over the following weeks, start replacing the least nutritious, processed foods with whole and fresh foods. You may find it easier to accomplish this one meal at a time or start by replacing one type of food, such as 'filler' snacks, with healthier alternatives. Over time, with practice and determination, it will become second nature to choose good foods over bad ones.
- While going through the above exercise, also note which foods are known triggers for your symptoms. When stomach ulcers are bleeding and you can't eat oranges without pain, why do you have oranges on your list? Listen to what your body is telling you and adjust accordingly.
- Note what you are drinking and how much clean water compared to alcohol, sodas, teas, coffees, etc. you are consuming.

- An elimination diet may be helpful to identify allergies or foods causing specific symptoms. Examples can be supported by a dietician.
- Experiment with new preparation methods, organic, whole foods, food combining, and juicing to add to your diet. It is no harder to buy fresh, organic foods when you know easy and fun preparation methods.
- Do some studying on natural nutritional supplements (do not take synthetic vitamins).
- Grow your own garden, make your own organic probiotics like kefir or kombucha, cook more meals at home, and include your family in the process. Adding the extra effort with the love it takes to provide and cook meals for yourself will make a difference in how you see your food.
- Be aware of the severity of current symptoms and make the decision to change your diet accordingly. Your health will get better and you will be able to eat some of those favorites you may not be able to today. Feeling deprived and agitated at what you can't eat doesn't support your emotional health. Instead, bask in the knowledge and be proud that you are helping your body to heal with every bite.
- Reduce sugar and replace it with honey or agave. This is one of the quickest ways to reduce inflammation and noticeable relief can be found within days. Watch food labels, as refined processed sugars are in ***everything*** pre-packaged and processed. (It is my belief that it is the only way to make processed, cardboard food palatable, so it goes without saying to stay away from processed foods, also.)

Developing your new lifestyle habits of how you think about eating is only difficult when you try to maintain the 'normal' eating habits you have grown accustomed to. You can redefine 'normal' to include foods that feed your cells with needed nutrition and foods that reduce inflammation with nontoxic alternatives. A new normal means reducing packaged breads, chips, fried foods, hot dogs, sodas, sugar-laden cereals and desserts, and just over-processed everything.

EAT TO FEED
FEEDING HEALTHY CELLS

With awareness of what you are actually eating, it becomes easier to replace the bad foods for good nutritious ones. Make a list of everything you eat for 14 days and note whether it is processed (P), whole (W), fresh (F) or filler (X) type. Add a nutritional value if you wish by using your intuition, also noting which foods are triggers for your symptoms. I recommend 14 days to get a full picture of what you eat and also how the foods react in your body. Use the following as a guide. If you are eating combined foods that include several ingredients, it is best to list them out such as a soup or taco or oatmeal with sugar and milk.

Food_____ Food_____
Type (P) (W) (F) or (X)_____ Type (P) (W) (F) or (X)_____
Nutritional value (1-3)_____ Nutritional value (1-3)_____
Symptom_____ Symptom_____

Food_____ Food_____
Type (P) (W) (F) or (X)_____ Type (P) (W) (F) or (X)_____
Nutritional value (1-3)_____ Nutritional value (1-3)_____
Symptom_____ Symptom_____

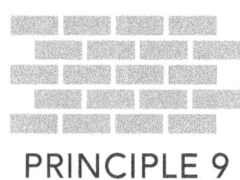

PRINCIPLE 9
GRATITUDE AND GRACE

Gratitude in times of struggle turns our toughest moments into steppingstones. See all as blessings.

It took me several years into my diagnosis before I could really be grateful for my symptoms and understand how to use that gratitude to help myself. Sitting in a church service one day listening to a sermon on gratitude, it struck home that this was a huge game changer—to just be happy despite everything. I am not sure that is where the minister was taking that message, but I saw things in a different light. I realized that I was trying to do the best I could but being very hard on myself in the process. Gratitude was a way to allow myself some grace; some happiness. As I relaxed into the feeling, I began to acknowledge the symptoms with thanks. I realized that it was my body's way (and maybe God's way) of telling me something was amiss in my pursuit of living my best life. In gratitude, I was able to react much more quickly to control the symptoms and do it with kindness for myself. It allowed me to sidestep the negative emotions of constantly feeling the victim or hateful for my disease. As I began to feel more gratitude towards myself, I also saw ways to be thankful for the people and their actions around me and developed a much more cheerful outlook toward life in general.

Humans are emotional creatures—it is what sets us apart from the rest of nature. Emotions stem from thoughts and reactions and create within us an attitude. In any given moment, about any given thing, we have an emotional reaction that in turn forms a thought or belief about the situation. We can use a belief to our benefit by creating a more cheerful attitude and then turning it into an action to support our healing process. The same holds true that a belief can hinder you from living your best life, keeping you in a stuck place of negativity and victimization.

Chronic illnesses can profoundly affect our emotions, evoking a wide range of feelings such as sadness, happiness, discontent, stress, contentment, anxiety, depression, grace, courage, and calmness. These emotions play a crucial role in managing our illness. Negative emotions often contribute to a sense of dis-ease, causing symptoms and affecting our health. Conversely, positive emotions can support the body's natural healing processes. Positive emotions make your body smile.

A good attitude can derail negative emotions that eventually wreak havoc with our immune system. I have found that there are several techniques to change our attitude for the better. Practicing patience and faith, building self-confidence, and looking at others with compassion are all things we would do well to develop. But the number one technique for getting your attitude in line with healing is practicing *gratitude.*

Gratitude is a state of being thankful and appreciating your blessings. It involves recognizing and valuing the positive aspects of your situation, leading to a greater sense of contentment and well-being.

Embracing gratitude for your disease symptoms, while initially may seem counterintuitive, can transform your well-being and your healing journey. By consciously acknowledging and blessing these symptoms, you shift from a mindset of resistance to one of acceptance and empowerment. By cultivating a mindset of gratitude, you can find meaning and determination even on the most challenging days, increasing inner peace and a deeper connection to your own strength.

We all have challenging days and obviously bad symptoms. Being grateful for those bad days and symptoms gave me the ability and the mindset to move forward to work on whatever was troubling me physically and emotionally. No one, not even your own body, wants to talk to someone who is angry or uncaring. Blessing your symptoms opens the door to listening to what your body is trying to tell you.

□□□

GIVING YOURSELF GRACE

Gratitude has an additional benefit to our lives that is often overlooked, and that is grace. Grace is understood as unearned divine favor or assistance, often seen as a special blessing. It can also mean to bestow honor or dignity. When you genuinely practice and embrace gratitude, you invite a sense of grace into your life. You bestow honor and dignity upon yourself. This grace will bring a calming peace and divine support that influences all your thoughts and actions, enriching both your own life and your interactions with others.

When you can make decisions from a place of grace and gratitude, not only will you do so with more clarity, but also with more strength and resilience. Just say thanks and ask, "What is my body trying to tell me?" then listen with grace for the answer.

> **Gratitude isn't just something you feel, it's a way of seeing the world. Grace is honoring that.**

HEALING HABIT 9: AN ATTITUDE OF GRATITUDE

Emotions to develop: Optimism, Passion
Emotions to be aware of: Entitlement, Jealousy

Gratitude takes you away from blame, anger, judgment, fear, and just about any other negative emotion you can think of. When you can honestly be thankful for not only the good things in your life and the people who you love, but also the challenges, pain, and discomfort or less-liked people, you support your body with the loving energy it thrives on.

- Bless conventional Western medicine. Say *out loud,* "Thank you for medications, doctors, and procedures for providing me with some relief."

  Realize that you need these things at this moment in your life and they are a gift. Hopefully, you will not always need to rely on them, but they are here for you now, so say thank you!

- Make a list of no less than twenty-five things you are grateful for in your life—big things, small things, and those you wouldn't ordinarily think to bless. Then, make this a daily ritual to add at least three things to be grateful for. Practicing gratitude in the moment is even more helpful.

- Discover in-depth specific things you are grateful for about your disease. This is a two-part process. First, list a very specific symptom you are experiencing currently, and then second, identify why you are grateful for that symptom. For example, your list may look like this:

Symptom: Diarrhea . . . thank you to my gut for alerting me to the fact that I have let my digestive tract reach such an inflamed state that it cannot function correctly and will cause me to be malnourished and dehydrated. *Or* thank you for reminding me that I need to deal with and release my anxiety in this situation.

Symptom: Aching joints and legs . . . thank you, nerves and muscles, for alerting me that my body is experiencing inflammation that it is fighting.

Symptom: Skin issues . . . thank you, skin, is there something that is an allergen to my body?

Symptom: Heart attack . . . thank you heart for helping me see relationship issues that may need to be addressed on an energetic level or a diet that needs detoxified.

- Spend a couple of minutes each day in prayer or meditation, feeling grateful for your life and accepting the grace that comes back to you. This practice can be combined with a current routine to create a new habit or as a focused activity.

It may be hard at first to bless your illness and its symptoms, but with practice you will be able to see that your body is just trying to help you be conscious of its problems. Bless your body and say thank you for the messages it is sending you. Respond with gratitude, and then be willing to do what it takes to fix the problem. Identifying a solution or a root cause will quickly become apparent while in a state of gratitude, and you will be able to make positive shifts for positive results.

> **I found a grace that I did not know was missing in taking care of myself.**

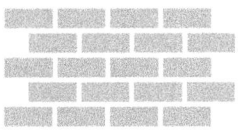

PRINCIPLE 10
TIME WELL SPENT

"He that can take rest is greater than he that can take cities."

–BENJAMIN FRANKLIN (POOR RICHARD'S ALMANACK, 1730S)

I remember when as a mom with Crohn's, I was determined to be a supermom—likely driven by a desire to defy my illness. I would often overdo things, and in my body's weakened state, I'd end up sleeping for hours or taking breaks on the couch. While it seemed that I was sometimes getting an overdose of rest, deep down, I wasn't okay with resting as much as I did or sleeping through half the weekend. Instead, I'd focus on how much I hated the disease, criticize myself for everything I hadn't accomplished, and feel guilty about the time I wasn't spending with my family. I resented the sleep my body needed to heal instead of being grateful for it. Over time, I realized there's a difference between simply resting or getting some sleep and allowing myself to truly relax and heal. When I let go and embraced rest as part of my self-care, a noticeable difference occurred.

In our modern over-achieving society, we overvalue productivity and undervalue sleep and relaxation. As a result, our bodies are very sleep- and rest-deprived. There is so much emphasis on being productive that taking time to rest can be considered wasted, and rest needed for healing is regarded as a personal failure. Scientists have extensively researched the connections between insufficient sleep and disease, and most experts have concluded that getting enough high-quality sleep is as important to health and well-being as nutrition and exercise. Sleep deprivation increases the levels of many inflammatory issues, and inflammation and infection in turn affect the amount and quality of sleep you get—creating a vicious cycle.

The first key point of this principle is your *attitude* about rest and sleep. You must give yourself *permission* to rest without guilt or feelings of failure. Resting when you need to rest is a self-care routine and habit to embody. Sleep provides the human body with the energy needed for cell rejuvenation and frees your mind from a constant barrage of never-ending thoughts. Bowing out of activities and getting the rest you need should never be thought of as selfish. If you are berating yourself for the amount of sleep you need today, know that with the healthier lifestyle habits you are developing, you will be able to do more as your body heals. But when you need rest, rest and be okay with it—and do it with a kind heart.

The second key point in this principle is to give yourself permission to do less and prioritize your time. Don't try to be the do-all and end-all of everything and everybody in your life. Let go of the super mom (or super dad) persona or the driven employee mindset. Prioritizing your time and efforts will not only result in a higher quality of life but will also take you out of the busyness that is an emotional and physical energy drain. By being more purposeful in how you spend your time, you can more easily include time for taking care of yourself.

OBLIGATIONS

Just like our modern world overvalues productivity, it is having quite an affair with obligation, too. We fill our calendars with endless tasks and duties, believing that conquering these commitments and responsibilities is the path to fulfillment. The pressure to constantly deliver—at work, at home, even in our personal thoughts—has slowly replaced the natural flow of creativity and well-being. We no longer allow ourselves the time to explore new ideas, follow our passions, or take care of our bodies until forced to; instead, we have become tied by the invisible cords of 'what must be done;' the 'have-to-dos.'

Many of the activities we engage in during the day are considered obligations; commitments we feel we 'have to' fulfill, whether by our own standards or a social norm. If your days are filled with activities that you feel are *required, resigned,* or *it is your duty* to do, your energy is being transferred to others—usually without reciprocation or appreciation. You may feel responsible, but your time and healing energy are being traded for the comfort of completing tasks, checking boxes, and meeting deadlines. If you are one who grinds through your obligations, it is time to really look at what that feels like in your body. When engaged in the activity, are you energized, anxious, or sighing heavily? Gaining a positive sense of accomplishment or just checking it off the list? As a rule, any activity that you feel obligated to do without choice will zap your physical and emotional energy quickly and is better limited, eliminated, or reframed.

Obligations can contribute to your wellbeing if done with an open heart and with the proper perspective. When you can reframe an activity as a desire to serve, personal growth, or purpose of accomplishment, then time spent on yourself, caring for and supporting family, religious practices, volunteering for social causes, or even work responsibilities becomes energy that promotes healing.

□□□

AIMS AND DESIRES

Aims and desires stem from your purpose and creativity. These are the things that inspire and excite you, fueling your energy and enthusiasm—your 'want-to-dos.' Passion and what you desire is the heart of personal expression and is the heart of what keeps life moving and worth living. Have you suddenly found an energy reserve you didn't realize you had when doing something you are passionate about? While you may tire quickly, the initial endorphin boost is noticeable, and these types of activities will raise your energetic and emotional vibration.

Different from obligations which satisfy a requirement or duty, aims and desires offer fulfillment and joy. Think of a desired activity as a picture where you see a smile on your face, your heart smiling, and your whole body right down to the foundational cells smiling, too. Smiling cells cannot stay diseased or ill for long.

Activities you are passionate about, such as making money or working, taking care of family, or completing school, can be either desires or obligations. The attitude we have while doing the activity or performing the task is the deciding factor. Turning obligations into desires is a mindset and can be accomplished by rethinking the activity. You will feel the difference in your body, and it is the goal to fill your days with as much of this positive, life-giving, creative energy as possible.

Smiling cells cannot stay diseased or ill for long.

SHOULDS

The word "should" is a guaranteed trigger for symptoms in our chronic illness world. Anything paired with 'should' can be removed from your life. Even thinking *I should take better care of myself* turns self-care into a burden—an obligation—rather than a desire. While 'should' can seem well-intentioned, it drains your energy by fueling anxiety, apprehension, and dread— negative emotions that weigh you down instead of lifting you up.

Just like how we see desires and obligations in light of the emotion they produce, thoughts and actions we have placed a 'should' in front of can also be reframed by seeing the activity from a different perspective. For example: you tell yourself you 'should' help your grandmother with cleaning her house, even though you are exhausted. In this moment, your mind is creating anxiety about what is now considered an obligation and gives you a feeling of dread. Instead, look at the activity as a gift by saying, "I am glad to have time with my grandmother, and I feel any amount of help I can give her is time well spent and good for both of us."

While you may still feel physically tired, this reframing fosters a more positive attitude toward what needs to be done.

How you label and view your time commitments can positively influence your emotions, transforming negativity into a more positive mindset. Your perspective on obligations, passions, aims, and desires either creates a healing space or negative emotions that feed your body's inflammatory response. Sometimes it is best to take action by purposefully doing nothing. And when you do take action, do it with purpose.

There's no greater waste than handling a task well when it shouldn't be done in the first place.

HEALING HABIT 10: PERMISSION TO DO—OR NOT

Emotions to develop: Respect, Enthusiasm
Emotions to be aware of: Resentment, Guilt

The idea of giving yourself permission to *rest* and then orchestrating the time to do so without guilt or a feeling of failure may feel ridiculous, daunting, or lifesaving, but when embraced, it is a game changer. Be honest as you go through this exercise and see how you can develop habits around rest. There are no right or wrong answers. Awareness will give you valuable insights into how your time is being spent and what changes are needed to help your body heal itself. Most of us have emotional and physical time and energy eaters that we do not realize have become routine habits in our lives. It is common when managing a chronic illness and you are not able to do the things you used to do to overcompensate, neglecting rest and healthy routines. Reclaim time for your rest and rejuvenation.

- Brainstorm a list of *all* the things you do during the day. Include everything from showering and personal care, watching your favorite TV show, doing laundry, phone calls and coffee dates, scrolling on social media, taking care of and playing with the kids or pets, eating, work and special projects, walking after dinner, hobbies, shopping, etc. Do this without judgment and listing everything with serious thought and honesty over a week's time. It may be helpful to make a ten-minute daily calendar and fill in those increments. As you brainstorm your activities, divide the list into two sections: *have-to-dos* and *want-to-dos*.
- Identify two or three items from the *have to do* list that are or

feel like obligations. Make a habit of analyzing each activity and note what that feels like in your body.

Are you energized or resigned with the activity? Gaining a sense of accomplishment or just checking it off the list?

Can you reframe the heaviest tasks to feel good when doing them by seeing each one as a gift of service?

Is there a way to transfer the task to another? An example might be to teach and organize family members to do the household chores to reduce your responsibility.

How can you eliminate the activity completely?

- Look at the tasks identified as *want-to-dos*. This list may be your self-care routines, your aims and desires, or your play time spent with friends and family. If you have a short list, be creative and fill in more fun, 'make you smile' activities that you would like to do. Try to make your *want-to-do* list at least as long as your *have-to-do* list.
- Go through your daily calendar and strive to replace at least 25 percent of the have-to-dos with want-to-dos. For example, if your mornings start with two hours of doing 'get out the door' tasks, you might replace thirty minutes of that time with a wakeup routine of taking fifteen minutes of setting the goals and tone for the day, and fifteen minutes to eat breakfast and enjoy focused time with a loved one. To reclaim those thirty minutes, it may take a few minutes the night before to make lunches or place items to easily grab by the door, but it will be well worth it for your peace of mind each morning.
- Get rid of all unnecessary time commitments. These may be on either the *have to* or *want to* list. It may take some time to decide which can stay and which can go and extract yourself

from some of those commitments but start by giving yourself permission to do so. Be ruthless and know that you are not irreplaceable. Women are notorious for not saying *no* when we really need to for a myriad of reasons. But men also need to look at the commitments that eat up their time and energy and cause anxiety around obligation or 'have-to-do.'

- Look at your *want-to-dos (aims and desires)* list one more time and identify any previous self-care routines that may be non-existent or haphazardly done now. It is time to purposefully schedule these in to make sure those are completed first. If your aim and/or desire is to help your body to heal and reduce symptoms, you also want to develop a habit that includes new or re-established self-care practices.

- Accept that even doing the *want-to-dos* are not always in your best interest. Give yourself permission to stay home and rest if that is needed. Trust that your family and friends want the best for you and will understand if you need to skip the family outing to sleep. Trust that things will get better, symptoms will lessen, you will have more energy, and you will be able to do the things you want to do. Patience with yourself is part of giving that permission to sleep, rest, and heal.

The goal for this healing habit is to become aware of what you spend your time on and if it is supporting your healing or supporting your disease. Time is our biggest commodity, and we can waste it or use it to our advantage. Give yourself permission to use your time wisely, and that includes giving your body the rest it needs to overcome the disease. Make some lifestyle choices that support your new decision.

TIME MANAGEMENT

Take a look at your Want-to-Do list. Are these really things you would like to do OR are they obligations that have eased themselves into 'should's'? A good way to tell the difference is by checking your excitement level. Things you really want to do will bring an excitement and a burst of energy & enthusiasm. The 'should's' will drain your energy before you start. Use your time wisely to create positives in your lifestyle to sustain healing.

These are should-do's I am going to release from my life ....
....
I want-to-do these things but I can wait until I am feeling better
....

Look at your Have-to-Do list and identify several activities that replaced with some extra rest. Think creatively how this can be accomplished. Can the kids make their own snacks? Can you hire some part time help for chores around the house? Can you take a bus or train to work? Think outside the box and reclaim some me time.

I can replace this obligation ....by doing this.....................
I can replace this obligation ....by doing this.....................
I can replace this obligation ....by doing this.....................

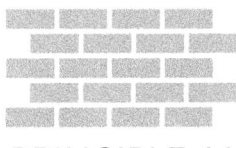

PRINCIPLE 11
A BODY IN MOTION

"A body in motion stays in motion; a body at rest stays at rest."
—SIR ISAAC NEWTON FIRST LAW OF MOTION

While I have never been a person who sits still for long, I am also not a physical exercise enthusiast. I am sure you can relate that when a disease is raging and every little movement hurts or the fatigue makes you motionless, exercise is the last thing on your mind. I found that I did not have to be a gym goer to get enough movement and exercise each day to keep my body healthy. I found it easy to stay in shape by engaging in chores, play, stretching, and doing a few sit-ups and push-ups, yoga, or walking each day. I also learned about some easy alternative treatments that included movement I could practice at home to target and support my immune system.

Our bodies are built to move, and this movement is a crucial foundation of good health. Exercise not only benefits the physical body but also our emotional and energetic health by producing stress-reducing hormones. A lack of exercise contributes to low self-esteem and causes your body to become stagnant and listless.

Some basic facts on muscle movement: as muscles contract, they play a crucial role in moving the liquids within our bodies, such as blood, lymph, and interstitial fluids. This rhythmic motion supports circulation by delivering oxygen and nutrients to tissues and organs and removes waste products. By keeping these fluids in motion, our muscles contribute significantly to the body's natural detoxification processes and the optimal functioning of our immune system. Muscle strength protects and supports our joints by reducing the risk of injury and improves mobility. Building and maintaining muscle through regular exercise and strength training is beneficial for improving metabolic health. This includes regulating blood sugar levels and stabilizing insulin levels, which supports long-term weight management and chronic illness management.

□□□

THE GYM OF LIFE

One of the common misconceptions of our modern society is that you need expensive equipment or physical trainers to achieve exercise, and this mindset even goes so far as to shame those not involved. Exercise can certainly include home gym equipment and memberships, but even easy movement like stretching, standing, walking, cleaning, gardening, or doing other chores is beneficial. Many of us have physically demanding jobs that suffice for exercise. In the case of someone battling chronic illness, these everyday activities are often more beneficial and easier on the body and mind than more structured routines. If you enjoy going to the gym and are able to do so, do it with enthusiasm and desire but do not restrict yourself from believing that it is the only way to adequately move your body. Create your exercise routine around what you enjoy doing and activities that create a sense of accomplishment—however large or small. Getting an adrenaline rush from walking with friends around the block or taking the dog for a run is sometimes all you need.

Understanding the basic foundation of movement and its importance to the body is key and worth developing habits around. Be intentional in developing habits that include some exercise.

□□□

HEALING HABIT 11: MOVE IT, GROOVE IT

Emotions to develop: Compassion, Enthusiasm
Emotions to be aware of: Guilt, Fear

Habits of consistent movement create a lifestyle where the body is constantly in a state of repair and renewal. Find ways each day to incorporate low-impact or small movements, as well as more aerobic exercises and strength training as tolerated. Know that any exercise is beneficial and that while you may be starting slowly, the intensity can increase as you feel ready. The key is to create a habit of keeping your body moving and energized and resist the tendency to become sedentary, blaming your illness.

Here are some easy ways to incorporate more movement into your lifestyle. Choose at least three to commit to daily:

- Stand up and stretch or walk around for a minute or two every hour, especially if you're sitting for long periods. These short breaks reduce stiffness and keep your energy levels up. Conversely, if you have a job that requires you to stand or move for extended periods of time, take breaks to shake out your legs and hands or sit down for a minute.

- Water exercises, whether in a pool or hot tub, can provide lower impact but high muscle use movement for a weakened body.
- Use the stairs instead of the elevator whenever possible for a quick way to increase your heart rate, move your joints, and add a little strength training.
- Choose a parking spot that's farther from the door so you can get a few extra minutes of walking in.
- Add quick exercises while at your desk, like seated leg lifts, shoulder rolls, or calf raises.
- Walking and playing with pets is great exercise and a good excuse to get out; playing tug-o-war with the dog is great for your upper body strength.
- Practice deep, diaphragmatic breathing by inhaling deeply through your nose, allowing your abdomen to expand, then exhaling fully. Repeat three to four times several times per day.
- A good massage not only moves energy in your body by releasing tension and emotions but also encourages lymph movement. You can practice self-massage techniques, focusing on areas like the neck, armpits, and groin to stimulate lymph nodes and hands, feet, lower back, and shoulders to release tension.
- Do household chores each day. Make your bed, do the laundry and dishes, and prepare meals. The benefits are two-fold by including movement and cleaning your space.
- Have a dance party with the little people in your world or grab your girlfriend and shake it out. Sing and move to a tune while cooking dinner, folding the laundry, in the shower, or in the carpool lane.
- SMILE! Using facial muscles is also an overall body, mind, and spirit boost!

PRINCIPLE 12

SETTING BOUNDARIES

Setting boundaries for yourself is one of the most loving things you can do.

I was my worst nightmare and often sabotaged my healthy efforts by doing things I knew were symptom-makers when I was feeling better. Whether it was eating something I knew I shouldn't (hot dogs and a beer seemed to be a must at a ball game when everyone else ordered the same) or taking on several new commitments with my newfound energy, or the processed foods and snacks that found their way back into the pantry, I often ignored my voice of reason. There was some therapeutic benefit to the occasional hot dog and beer, but when I too easily slid back into old habits and routines, I realized I needed a way to counteract that all too human tendency. I learned to set some boundaries for myself to never (or rarely) cross. While I still have my days that I do things I know aren't in my best interest, I am much better at staying within the boundaries I set for myself. This is especially true when opting for rest, spending time in nature, my self-care routines, and taking supplements that support and enhance my health. I found that it is much easier to make decisions in the moment when there is a line I have already decided I will not cross.

Setting boundaries is like building a sturdy fence around a well-tended garden—it protects what matters most and creates a space for growth. By clearly defining your limits, you establish a foundation that nurtures healthy habits and prevents distractions or harmful influences from creeping in. Boundaries should not be thought of as barriers but acts of self-respect and self-care that allow you to say "yes" to what helps you heal and "no" to what detracts from it. These are the spectrum of practices that you will stay within to hold yourself accountable and are the lines not to cross when you *know* it will cause a symptom or sabotage your efforts in helping your body heal.

Holding to your boundaries to keep from backsliding will be an aspect of those moment-to-moment decisions you make. Develop a habit to listen to your intuition and decide when it is best to stay within your boundaries. The key is to establish the foundational framework and have it ready when needed.

ㅁㅁㅁ

LIFESTYLE ENHANCERS

Lifestyle enhancers are more than just indulgences; they are intentional acts that replenish your energy, soothe your mind, and strengthen your body's ability to heal. These practices improve not only your physical health but also your emotional and mental well-being. By protecting these lifestyle enhancers with firm boundaries—whether it's scheduling them into your routine or saying "no" to commitments that interfere—you ensure they remain a consistent part of your life. This commitment to have boundaries reinforces the connection between self-care and your body's remarkable capacity to heal itself.

FOLLOWING THE CROWD

I mentioned earlier how our environment plays a major role in the habits we adopt, and it is important to revisit this concept when talking about boundaries. Habits and behaviors are developed in large part by the people you hang out with or identify with most. This can be a disadvantage, as social norms are easy to follow. It can be challenging to eat healthier when others around you are still eating processed, packaged foods, or if you wish to work fewer hours and there is an expectation to work more in your company. By creating a boundary around what is best for you, you protect your healing efforts.

You can also use this concept of environment and social norms to your advantage by making sure those around you support your efforts of healing. If your office has a fitness campaign, then participating will provide you with accountability. It is easier to believe an idea is doable and real when others are also on the same path. The key is to develop habits that allow you to stay within your boundaries, not to buck the crowd and create that healing environment. Surround yourself with like-minded people, supporters that you can also support.

All of the realizations, knowledge, and choices you make to keep yourself healthy come down to the boundaries you set and the ability to stand your ground.

HEALING HABIT 12: THE LINES NOT TO CROSS

Emotions to develop: Confidence, Determination
Emotions to be aware of: Insecurity, Guilt, Unworthiness

To maintain your sustainable, healthy lifestyle habits, the time to set boundaries is when you are not feeling as healthy as you would like. While your symptoms are lessened but still bothering you, it is a perfect time to decide how to make them not come back. You do not want to fall into the cycle of: you feel well, forgetting everything you have been doing to help yourself, and then backsliding and having to start all over.

Have you ever felt better for months and have decided that you can take that extra class or two at college and suddenly you fall victim to the anxiety of getting all As? Or you find that you are eating a hotdog at each home baseball game you attend and are wondering why your heartburn is back? Or maybe you have taken a new job, and with its new time commitments, you find yourself eating nothing but fast food. Or a common reaction when you have been symptom-free for an extended length of time is to have your friends, family, and/or spouse start making demands on you that they didn't before. They 'forget' that you have a disease and may start expecting more of your time and energy.

Think of this as a linear ruler, with one end of the spectrum being set boundaries that will help you to say no to things that you *may* at one point think you feel well enough to do (starting with one as absolute nos). These are the life activities or situations that you know will cause symptoms, inflammation, or throw your emotions off balance. On the opposite end of the spectrum (ten) are your lifestyle enhancers. The absolute yesses are the things you do to specifically to take care of yourself, calm your nerves, and help your body heal.

THE ABSOLUTE NOS

Spend some serious thought about what lines you *will not* cross going forward to maintain your health and healing. These will be your absolute nos. Developing this habit is a powerful exercise, and it will give you confidence, determination, and ground to stand on when the issue needs to be faced, as it eventually will at some point.

Examples of some NO boundaries and lines not to cross you may set are:

- Limit or never eat the specific foods that are known triggers or allergens for you.
- Not eating foods or using products for personal care that have known carcinogens listed on the label.
- Not volunteering for more than one organization at a time to concentrate your efforts and not create a situation where you are overwhelmed.
- Striving to put yourself first when it comes to your energy allowance.
- Not being a doormat that makes you feel unappreciated.
- Not letting others coerce you into eating something or doing an activity that at the time is not in your best interest just to save face.
- Limiting time spent in relationships that are demeaning, abusive, or unsupportive.
- Not biting off more than you can chew with time commitments or desires that require you to give up self-care practices, such as going back to work or school full time.

As you establish these lines you are unwilling to cross, feel the strength and pride in yourself that comes with loving and supporting the decision to help yourself.

◻◻◻

THE ABSOLUTE YESSES

Now think about some specific habits or practices that are your life enhancers—your absolute yesses. (Be sure you have given yourself permission to treat and support yourself without any guilt.)

- Start by listing the life enhancers that you will always want to include in your life. They may be a part of your core values and are just needed to make your life complete, or they may be things that bring you physical or emotional comfort. Some examples are time in nature, nurturing relationships with loved ones, volunteer opportunities, time with friends, a cozy reading day, and alternative treatments. These can change, expand, or be irrelevant at different times, so treat this as a continual working list.
- Other lifestyle enhancers you want to make a habit of can be:
Therapeutic Massage: Massage is not just about relaxing muscles—even though this is a *great* way to relieve tension, stress, and anxiety. A good therapist will be able to move energy around in the body and release many of the physical and emotional traumas and toxins that have collected in it and are now a root cause of your disease. Set up a recurring appointment that you do not have to think about and are able to make a routine habit.

Research and New Knowledge: Stay abreast of current, good, unbiased research being done in conventional medicine and holistic and alternative healing treatments. Concise knowledge that can be used as the situation warrants is good to have. Never stop learning about your disease, but do not dwell on it either.

Alternative Therapies: Body work such as Reiki, acupuncture, sound therapy, essential oils, and nature bathing are some examples of alternative therapies that have all been found to be viable treatments for chronic illness. The list is getting longer each day as the world embraces more natural holistic treatments.

Self-Development Courses: We are all on a different path and in a different place in our self-development. There are so many good healers and self-development books that can give you just the insight you need. The goal here is to create a fulfilling, happy life that is free from disease. Make a habit to develop a better you.

Life Coach: Someone to help you navigate through the emotional traumas and lifestyle changes you desire to change is invaluable. This disease will leave scars not only in your body but in your emotional health as well, so find a third-party advocate who supports you.

Lifestyle enhancers will be a huge blessing in your life going forward, not only as a way to control symptoms and help your body to heal, but also to empower your life force—both for yourself and others.

THE LINES NOT TO CROSS
BOUNDARIES

What you allow is what will continue so setting boundaries is an important step to maintaining your hard- earned decisions you make to sustain your healthy lifestyle.

Physically and Emotionally we all need personal boundaries in place. Make your list as to what lines you will not cross going forward to maintain your health and healing.

The Lines not to Cross:
I refuse to allow……………………………………………………………
I refuse to allow……………………………………………………………
I refuse to allow……………………………………………………………
I refuse to allow……………………………………………………………
I refuse to allow……………………………………………………………

My Lifestyle Enhancers:
I will always…………………………………………………………………
I will always…………………………………………………………………
I will always…………………………………………………………………
I will always…………………………………………………………………
I will always…………………………………………………………………

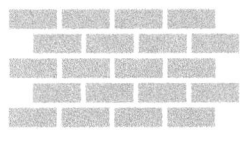

PRINCIPLE 13

CRAVINGS, IMPULSES, AND ADDICTIONS

"Impulses are often the echoes of our inner conflicts; they shout louder when we try to ignore them."

—UNKNOWN

Something I called my 'guilty pleasure' when doing the mom 'drop-off and pick-up' routine was to drive through the new coffee kiosk and pick up a large mocha latte. I loved that first taste of hot chocolatey goodness! It would usually cause a reaction in my gut, and I would be mad at myself for having indulged in something I knew would hurt me. In my anger created from feeling the victim, I justified that it was my guilty pleasure and damn the disease. Begrudgingly, I had a 'heart to heart' talk and came to terms with why I was torturing myself with, of all things, a bought coffee. Seeing my guilty pleasure not as the reward I believed it was, but an impulse buy that was coming from a place of overwhelm, I improved a habit or two to stay ahead of my schedule. It wasn't the mocha latte I needed so much as the comfort of doing something for myself and indulged in to erase the overwhelm I was feeling. I found an alternative to the dairy-filled, sugar laden chocolate coffee that was a sure-fire symptom producer and started a healthier habit of taking care of and indulging myself.

Cravings, impulses, and addictions are the body's way of signaling unmet needs, unresolved emotions, or imbalances. We need not go deep into the psychology of these behaviors here, but it is important to become aware of how they fit into and affect our healing lifestyle. These behaviors often mask deeper wants of connection, relief, or nourishment, and while they can feel overpowering, they are not the enemy—they are messages inviting us to pause, listen, and respond with curiosity instead of judgment.

Addictions such as drugs, smoking, drinking, and overeating the wrong foods are even more pronounced and physically unhealthy due to the struggle your body goes through daily. These are things to either stop completely or do in moderation. I trust (since this is true of most people) that at some point in your life, you have either already accomplished giving up an addiction or are well aware you need to stop doing something. If you have beaten an addiction, it is a success you should celebrate. If you know you need to stop, now is the time.

Whether you gave up the addiction because you had to (hard to smoke in the hospital or overeat when food makes you ill) or it was a choice you made and succeeded in, realize that you did this to *take care of you*. You already know the drill and know that it can be accomplished, so there is no need to carry any addictions forward. If you feel you need support in your addiction, please go back to the lifestyle enhancers and include this as a need to get help with. The decision to take the steps needed to stop any bad habits that have become addictions will serve you well.

Cravings often stem from both emotional and physical responses, frequently triggered by a sense of deprivation or imbalance. Cravings for food can signal a nutritional deficiency, indicating the body's need for specific nutrients or on an emotional level, and may come from feelings such as stress, loneliness, or dissatisfaction, as food is often associated with comfort and reward. Recognizing the root cause of cravings is essential to managing them effectively. By pausing to assess what is being craved and why, it becomes possible to make choices that align with your overall well-being. If a craving serves a positive purpose—whether it's addressing a nutritional gap or providing a sense of enjoyment—do it with the awareness of the positive effect it is creating.

Impulses tend to originate from being out of control, unfocused, or overwhelmed with stress. It is a desire that in the moment you think will make you feel better either emotionally or physically. In these moments, the urge to reach for a quick fix stems from a desire to soothe discomfort or fill an emotional void. Much like my mocha latte habit, these decisions can become symbolic of surrendering control, which can derail the healthy lifestyle habits you are striving to develop. While it may provide a temporary sense of relief or reward, thechoices we make on impulse often have long-term consequences, leaving us feeling worse physically and emotionally unempowered.

□□□

REDIRECTING YOUR FOCUS

The key to managing addictions, cravings, and impulses lies in cultivating awareness and redirecting your focus. When the urge strikes, pause and ask yourself what your body or mind truly needs. Is it nourishment, rest, or perhaps emotional comfort? Instead of giving in to the unhealthy response, replace it with positive action. This positive action will allow you to distance yourself so that you can stop and listen to what your body (or mind) is trying to tell you. Over time, training yourself to choose alternatives that support your well-being strengthens your self-discipline and reinforces your healthy habits. Remember, every small, mindful choice keeps you on the path to balance and helps prevent the downward spiral that can sabotage your progress. Use the healing principles as a structure to develop the foundational habits to stand on to feel empowered and happier with yourself.

> *"I count him braver who overcomes his desires than him who conquers his enemies; for the hardest victory is over self."*
>
> —ARISTOTLE

HEALING HABIT 13: TAMING THE BEAST WITHIN

Emotions to develop: Hopefulness
Emotions to be aware of: Insecurity, Guilt, Unworthiness

Be in control of your wants, desires, cravings, impulses, and addictive behaviors by identifying how these emotions and actions affect your body. Do not use your disease or bad habits and choices to justify either one or the other.

- Make a list of the craving, impulse, or addictive behaviors that may be causing some of your symptoms or you know are triggers but you do anyway. Ask yourself why and what you are getting out of it? Are there healthier choices you can make to help yourself not to feel deprived or out of control? Do you need a counselor or coach to help you with the issue? There are no right or wrong answers here; just awareness is what we are seeking.

- If you have a behavior you are trying to overcome, research has found that replacing it with a positive habit is the most effective way to stop and redirect your actions. While not always easy, this can be accomplished with a simple three-step process:

  1. First, identify the behavior you wish to eliminate.

  2. Identify a positive action you can replace it with.

  3. Attach this new action to an already established habit.

  Examples of positive actions could be stopping to take three deep breaths, calling a friend, drinking a glass of water, reaching for a wholesome snack, starting a hands-on activity such as doing the dishes, or taking a short walk.

Establishing a mindful relationship with cravings, impulses, and addictions fosters both control and satisfaction, preventing feelings of restriction that can lead to a cycle of overindulgence. Addressing these actions thoughtfully may include small, intentional allowances, or stopping completely. By understanding your reasons, it becomes possible to maintain balance between physical health and emotional fulfillment.

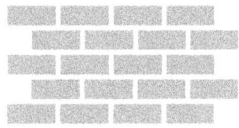

PRINCIPLE 14

THE LAW OF ATTRACTION

"For it is in giving that we receive."

—ST FRANCIS OF ASSISI

I have often commented in jest that I would be a rich woman if I had a nickel for every hour I have volunteered over the years. But truth be told, it was all time I enjoyed, even though it was at times more effort than I could physically handle. Volunteering provided me with a sense of connection and community that was outside my health issues, and I felt more normal, accepted, and accomplished, which helped my attitude and also filled me with positive purpose and energy. Even though I was not thinking specifically about how my volunteer service was affecting my health over the years, looking back I see that it was one of those game changers. I am indeed a rich woman for the time I gave freely, but I believe without a doubt that it is a major reason why I am healthy today.

The law of attraction teaches us that our thoughts and emotions shape our reality, whether that outcome is staying stuck in a negative, woe-is-me state or empowering us to take an active role in our own health and well-being. Simply stated, the law of attraction says, "like attracts like," or "what you think about you get."

By focusing on positive outcomes and believing in our body's ability to heal, we align ourselves with energy that supports not only recovery but sustainable healing.

□□□

THE POWER OF GOODWILL

One of the easiest and most profound ways to create a feeling of well-being is to give to others. Acts of service—such as volunteering, supporting a cause, or simply offering kindness—shift our focus from internal struggles to outward connection, giving us a sense of purpose and helping us to recognize the strength and value we possess. When we engage in acts of kindness and generosity, it triggers the release of 'feel-good' hormones like oxytocin and endorphins, which will provide a shift in our emotional state, reducing stress, anxiety, and feelings of isolation—all of which have been determined to be significant barriers to healing.

In a world that frequently prioritizes productivity in measurable achievements, tangible outcomes, and individual success, the quiet, behind-the-scenes power of goodwill can be overlooked or undervalued. These acts of kindness, generosity, and compassion positively reinforce the belief that we are contributors to our own lives and the lives of others. Feed your passions and your body by serving in that capacity.

Goodwill is a powerful yet understated tool for aligning our emotional and physical health on the path to healing. Acts of service to others help us to counteract the negative energy of hopelessness or fear that a self-focused, victim-oriented mindset creates, and instead gives us a sense of purpose, connection, and belonging. Goodwill also promotes mutual exchange; when we give to others, we often receive support, encouragement, and care in return, creating a cycle of positivity that enhances our lives.

In your journey to support your body's healing, focusing constant worry on your illness and its symptoms can unintentionally draw more of the same—more discomfort and challenges. Dwelling on thoughts like, *I have a diseased body, I'm always so exhausted,* or *no one understands me* only serves to sustain a cycle that impacts your mental, emotional, and physical well-being. By shifting your focus toward nurturing thoughts, you can create an environment where healing becomes not just possible but inevitable.

> *"The best way to find yourself is to lose yourself in the service of others."*
>
> –MAHATMA GANDHI

□□□

HEALING HABIT 14: POWER IN GIVING

Emotions to develop: Accomplishment, Enthusiasm
Emotions to be aware of: Unworthiness, Powerlessness

Shift your focus away from your symptoms and personal struggles and instead embrace caring for others, finding joy in connections and purpose, and being of service. What you focus on expands, and by concentrating on compassion and contribution, you invite more of those generous feelings into your life. Start small—practice daily habits like expressing gratitude, offering help to a friend, or volunteering for a cause that resonates with you. These intentional actions not only benefit others but also create a ripple effect of healing and well-being within yourself.

- The law of attraction encourages you to pay attention to your thoughts. Take time to write down the strongest or most recurring thoughts you have during the day. (An average person has over 10,000 thoughts per day.) Acknowledging where most of these thoughts come from and the feelings attached to them will help you understand how you need to pivot your focus. For example:

    Fear of Failure: If you often think, *I'll never succeed*, it may stem from past experiences where you felt inadequate or did not have success in something you tried. Recognizing this can help you shift your focus to your achievements, however small, and cultivate a mindset of growth and resilience instead of dwelling on past disappointments.

    Self-Criticism: Thoughts like *I'm not good enough* might come from societal standards or a comparison to others. Acknowledging this influence allows you to turn towards self-compassion, reminding yourself of your unique strengths and the value you bring, fostering a healthier self-image.

    Embracing Change: If you find yourself thinking *what if things go wrong?*, this might be rooted in a fear of the unknown. Recognizing this can encourage you to focus on the potential for positive outcomes and opportunities for growth, embracing change as a chance for new experiences rather than a threat.

- Look again at your core values and then list your skills to help identify where you could be of service to others or in your community. For example, I had a core value of nurturing my children, was skilled at organizing and teaching, and liked the outdoors. Combining the three, I was able to provide years of service to outdoor youth organizations and teaching programs.
- Identify an organization or causes you can become passionate about being involved in.
- Reach out to people you can help and support and who provide you with good positive interaction like good neighbors needing assistance.
- Service to others needs to become an important commitment on that 'want-to-do' list.

Remember to perform service with passion and with joy of giving. Do not do it from a place of 'should' or out of obligation. Also, going overboard to the point of exhaustion and feeling overwhelmed defeats the purpose. It is not always easy to participate if you are not feeling well, so pick something that you can enjoy with little or a variable time commitment. Doing for others is doing for you. Make it an outpouring of loving support so that it becomes one of your reasons to be healthy and a part of your life purpose.

> **It is impossible to feel sadness when making another smile. It is impossible to feel discouraged about your own journey when focused on building another up. It is impossible to be angry when making someone laugh. It is impossible to feel useless when providing a valued service to others.**

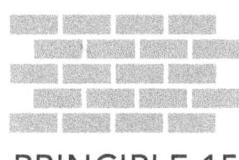

PRINCIPLE 15
ROUTINES AND RHYTHMS

*"We are what we repeatedly do.
Excellence, then, is not an act, but a habit."*

–ARISTOTLE (4TH CENTURY BC, NICOMACHEAN ETHICS)

When I was a child, I had a great-grandmother who was raised to be prim and proper, brought up in the early 1900s. She also exuded a strength of purpose that was rooted in her routines that I remember to this day. Her schedule was filled with social events, volunteerism, and shopping—'being out,' as she called it. Her routine in the morning could be timed to the minute of getting up with the sun, making a cup of black tea, fixing a piece of toast, and then getting herself 'presentable' for her day. I remember feeling ill one morning when I was at her house. As I lay there on the couch and talked to the doll I had (no TV, as that was reserved for the evening), she asked me why my hair was not combed or I had not gotten out of my 'night clothes.' (Being all of five years old, I am guessing it was because no one had told me to yet and I had no place to go I knew of.)

Without a second thought, I was herded off to the bath to clean up and put on some 'day clothes,' and with the excitement of thinking we were going out, I had a bit more energy. There was no going out that day, and I spent it still laying on the couch 'tending' my fever (except for sitting on the front porch for ten minutes to get some fresh air and sun). I asked her, while getting back into my 'night clothes' before bed that night, why I had needed to even get dressed that day. Her matter-of-fact answer was that "it makes you feel better." That act of getting up, washing my face, combing my hair, and getting dressed was so impactful that to this day, despite illness, being up all night with my pain or crying babies, working from home, or any other reason I might wake up not wanting to start my day, I will, at some point, clean up, put myself together, and (whether or not I will be going out) put on my 'day clothes.'

Routines are intentional, repeated actions or habits that we create to bring structure and predictability to our daily lives. They can be extensions of natural rhythms and tend to make us feel connected and comfortable. Routines add a sense of security, stability, and confidence to a healing environment that can provide relief from managing too many thoughts. When we are detoured from a normal routine, it can bring on either subtle anxiety or a serious undoing of our life.

There are very few days that go by that something, given the opportunity, won't disrupt your schedule or security, igniting that fight-or-flight reaction. Small interruptions can go by unnoticed for a while but will compound over time. Larger challenges such as managing a disease, taking care of a newborn, starting college or a new job, or caring for a child or parent are easier to notice. All interruptions can put your life into a tailspin (if only for a moment before you regain control), but with awareness and effort, you can reestablish a routine around the issue. Routines can take a haphazard schedule of chaotic thoughts and spur-of-the-moment or rushed actions to a more tranquil, thought-out lifestyle. Calmly develop routines that support your body in its healing during these times and they become a sustainable lifestyle habit.

Healthy personal routines are tools that are easy to develop. While it can help mentally to create routines for getting to work, the kids up and to school, consistent meal times, and the like, routines that *personally support you* such as a weekly yoga class or meditation and journaling in the morning to start your day can have a tremendous impact on your healing journey. Be aware of easily developed routines that are counter-productive and can derail your healthy habits, such as skipping meals, sitting for long periods, whether at a desk or on the couch, poor sleep habits, too much screen time, or mindless snacking during work breaks.

Routines that are done regularly become habits and are one of the more sustainable ways to bring our body back into balance.

□□□

INTUITIVE PATTERNS

Rhythms are natural, intuitive patterns that align with your body's needs and the cycles of nature. At our core, humans have a strong connection to nature and this affects us at a deep unconscious level, such as when we feel tired when it's dark or when we crave warmth in winter.

The natural rhythms of ocean waves, full moons, seasonal changes, and the rising and setting of the sun give us a foundation for tuning into the natural balance of life. The body follows several natural rhythms, which work to create harmony with our environment that when allowed, support a deeper connection to yourself and a way to balance basic functions. The circadian cycle is our body's natural twenty-four-hour rhythm, which regulates essential functions like sleep, energy levels, and digestion. Metabolic rhythms regulate heartbeats, breathing, and hormone levels as needed. Working with our natural rhythms can enhance our energy and well-being. It is how the body is designed.

A disease will affect many of the body's rhythms, and to help your body heal, it helps to pay attention to daily patterns and re-align with the natural rhythms. When we embrace the gentle natural rhythms, such as waking with the sunrise and sleeping after sunset or eating when hungry, we give the body the natural space it needs, reducing stress and allowing it to restore, repair, and renew itself. This leads to not only a more balanced life but is one of the best ways to accomplish our small improvements towards healing. I have found this is one of the easiest ways to help your body.

> **Our daily routines shape the environment in which the body heals, turning small, consistent actions into powerful pathways to wellness. When we embrace the gentle rhythms, we give the body the space it needs to restore, repair, and renew itself.**

□□□

HEALING HABIT 15: BACK INTO RHYTHM

Emotions to develop: Contentment, Security
Emotions to be aware of: Insecurity, Anxiety

Recognize if you have given up any of your personal routines or ignored any natural rhythms while managing the symptoms of your disease since being diagnosed. You need to be intentional in incorporating as many structured routines in your day as you can and do so using natural rhythms to bring order and balance to your life.

- **Connect with nature by noticing the current season and how that looks and feels.**

    Rhythm: Spend time outside during sunrise, sunset, or other calming moments when nature's rhythms are most evident.

    Routine: Schedule daily or weekly nature walks or outdoor time to stay connected.

- **Nourish your body as needed.**

    Rhythm: Eat in tune with your hunger and fullness.

    Routine: Plan balanced meals in advance to ensure you're meeting your nutritional needs, drink water before each meal, eat at the same time each day, and practice intermittent fasting.

- **Develop a morning routine to set the tone of the day.**

    Rhythm: Wake up naturally with the sunrise or as your body feels ready.

    Routine: Start your day with a consistent practice, such as journaling, stretching, a morning meditation, or making a short list of to-dos.

- **Develop a sleep routine.**

    Rhythm: Align your sleep schedule with your body's natural tiredness and the day-night cycle.

    Routine: Create a nightly wind-down ritual like reading, stretching, or sipping herbal tea.

- **Movement and exercise release endorphins and other healthy chemicals.**

Rhythm: Choose activities that match your energy levels, such as yoga on low-energy days or a brisk walk when you feel energetic.

Routine: Schedule specific times to exercise regularly to maintain consistency.

- **Recognize times of productivity at work.**

    Rhythm: Pay attention to your focus and energy peaks, such as morning productivity versus afternoon lull, and plan tasks accordingly.

    Routine: Set fixed times for work with scheduled breaks. Leave work at work as much possible.

- **Prioritize self-care practices.**

    Rhythm: Tune into when you feel you need to nurture yourself, like after a stressful day, and respond to rather than ignore your needs.

    Routine: Dedicate a specific time weekly to a self-care ritual, like a long bath, a creative hobby, or taking a personal day.

- **Tune into your body.**

    Rhythm: Use breathing exercises as you calm your body, your mind, and your emotions as you ask and then listen to what your body is saying.

    Routine: Use automatic notifications on meditation apps and soft music to prompt a routine to stop, breathe, and listen.

- **Address routines that have become unhealthy habits and replace them with a more sustainable option.**

Routines offer discipline and accountability in consistent practice, and rhythms invite you to listen to the connection of your body and nature. Each is an important tool in our healing and will create a structure that will enhance all of the other principles.

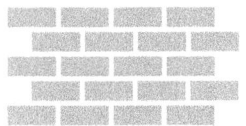

PRINCIPLE 16
HEALING SPACES

*"And into the forest I go,
to lose my mind and find my soul."*

–JOHN MUIR

I spent much of my life living in the city, where it was easy to work and be in a neighborhood that supported friendships and community for the family. We also spent many hours involved in out-of-town activities that included hiking, weekend camping, and summer camps. While it was a herculean effort most times to get all of the food and gear together, I looked forward to being out among nature, sleeping on the ground, and enjoying the elements. I admit I am a nature person and know I need those elemental connections, but didn't appreciate why until years later. I found I felt best when in communion with anything outdoors or nature related. It calms my nerves, my body, and my thoughts. While I love the energy of a city full of productivity and people, after a while, I feel stifled and anxious about too much concrete and contained space. I learned to soothe my anxiety with sojourns into the outdoors.

The energy of the communities around you, the people you spend time with, and even the information you consume, as we have seen, all play a significant role in defining who you are. We have talked about how your environment influences your thoughts, habits, and behaviors, and to succeed in sustaining new habits, your surroundings must align with your desired outcome. It is important for you to also understand how the spaces you spend the most time in—usually your home, your office, and/or outdoors—play a significant but often unappreciated role in our healing.

□□□

NATURE AS HEALER

Making a habit of spending time in nature is a simple routine to enhance your healing process. Being in a natural environment will calm your nerves, realign your natural rhythms, boost your mood, reduce stress, and balance your energy, making it, in my opinion, a non-negotiable healthy lifestyle habit for anyone managing disease. Some specific ways nature can boost your health include:

- Natural sounds such as flowing water and chirping birds promote relaxation and reduce stress.
- Being outdoors encourages physical movement like hiking or walking on the beach or through the park and gives all the benefits of increased immune function that exercise provides.
- Mindfulness and calming emotions and thoughts can be achieved by being present in nature by simply noticing the flowers or feeling connected to the bigger picture of a vista, sunrise, or sunset.
- Soaking up a healthy dose of vitamin D from the sun and breathing fresh air are both natural immune boosters.

- The science and research being published about grounding (walking barefoot, sitting, or lying on the earth) is compelling in describing the reconnection of the body's frequency with the Earth's and how that promotes emotional balance and reduces inflammation.
- The emotional and heart connection to something greater than ourselves can reduce anxiety and produce chemicals that relax the body.

As mentioned in our rhythms and routines principle, we as humans are deeply connected to nature whether we realize it or not, so it serves you well to create times and places that speak to you where you can make this natural connection. Do not discount this all-important aspect of your being and the natural holistic treatment it can provide.

□□□

CLEARING THE INSIDE CLUTTER

I have always been a re-arranger of the furniture, decorations, and cabinets or routinely cleared out spaces that seemed to get too full of 'things' left lying around (or stacked up in the corners to be dealt with later). While I am not considered OCD by any means and never had a home so organized or pristine to be on a magazine cover, I would go on a routine cleaning and clearing rampage when the clutter seemed to overwhelm me to the point of a physical attack on my system. This activity seemed to put my world and emotions back in order. I found myself craving healing spaces and environments without really knowing that was my point.

The space you live and work in says a lot about your life, so design your indoor office and home spaces in ways that provide calmness and rejuvenation to your body and spirit. Creating a healing atmosphere at home and/or work will boost your energy and support your body to heal itself. The power of a space that feels aligned with who you are is invaluable to support your good health. When you feel the space around you is comforting, alive with possibility, clean, clear, and energized, your body will feel the same. Surround yourself with fun, creative, exciting, efficient, and comforting things. Make your environment reflect the healthy person you wish to be.

If you are living in a space crammed with old, unused things, dead plants, and devoid of beauty or comforting articles, you will hold those same energies in your body. These overwhelming spaces will drain your energy and leave you depressed and exhausted. The space around you is a direct reflection of your body and inner emotions.

As I discovered in my cleaning, clearing, and purifying rampages, it put my emotions and energy back into a healthy balance and put my world in order. It wasn't just about the physical disarray of the house, but rather the stagnant energy that made it hard to focus and feel in control. Energy in our spaces can be felt, and each of us have some of these types of examples in our lives. You may, for instance, remember a time when you were searching for a new home and as you walked into different possibilities, the vibe just wasn't right. And then, after finding the perfect place and moving in, the feeling of newness it provided made you smile with excitement and possibilities. It is even likely that much of the furniture and items you meticulously packed and moved didn't fit well into the new space. That is because they didn't! There is a beautiful, unique energy when we can start fresh, releasing the old and making way for the new.

If you have lived or worked in the same space for years, clearing old items from your home, office space, and even computer will prove invaluable to you in ways you may never be consciously aware of. Letting go of unused or unnecessary items symbolizes releasing old habits, beliefs, or emotions that no longer serve you. With just a small amount of cleaning and clearing, you allow positive, healthier new energy to enter. Strive to create fresh new spaces that your thoughts, attitudes, and energies can thrive in to empower your healing lifestyle.

> **Anywhere your body, mind, and soul can feel comfortable and energized is a healing space.**

□□□

HEALING HABIT 16: SPACE TO HEAL

Emotions to develop: Peaceful, Calm
Emotions to be aware of: Boredom, Motionless

Getting out into nature, even for short bursts of time, will help the body to heal not only physically but mentally, as well. Spend sixty to ninety minutes minimum outdoors each day, breaking up the time and activity as needed.

- Spend twenty minutes in the sun (even if it's cloudy).
- Let the raindrops or snowflakes hit your face for a minute or two; the childlike delight will see you smiling.
- Walk outside after dinner or at lunch. If you live in the city, search for parks and open spaces to walk through and enjoy.
- Drive to an overlook and embrace the vista.
- Schedule time to watch the sunrise or sunset, taking deep breaths and taking in the grandeur of the scene. Or step

outside and just take a few deep breaths while you look up at the sky.
- As often as possible, take a drive to the outskirts of town and enjoy the change of scenery. Notice the seasons.
- Connect to the natural elements of fire, water, air, and earth each day.
- Candles can be used during meditation and to clear stagnant energies in your spaces.
- Open the windows if you can and let the fresh breeze in to move stagnant energy out.
- Fountains can be connections to water and small ones are easy to add to an indoor living space.
- Bring nature in by having houseplants, an herb garden, or fresh flowers inside your home.
- Collect or buy crystals, rocks, or other outdoor treasures to display.

In the Home: Look around the place you spend the most time in. Cleaning, clearing, and freshening the space can be done in small steps. Notice your emotions as you identify things around your home and take steps to feel better in these spaces. Some examples are:
- Are the countertops overflowing with things that need to be thrown away, washed, or put away? Make a habit of spending ten minutes to clean up daily.
- Are there unread magazines lying around you haven't read yet?
- Are there clothes in your closet from ten to twenty years ago that you know should go?
- Is your basement or attic stuffed full of boxes that have not been opened in years?

- Do your windows need to be washed or repaired?
- Is there broken furniture, unfinished projects, or is the room itself in disrepair?
- Choose objects to bring into your home that nurture your spirit.
- How can you bring some nature in? Plants, fountains, crystals, nature scenes (either real or in beautiful pictures), and photos can add comfort.
- How can you create a place to snuggle into where you can become your most peaceful and energetic, alive self? What feeds your soul?
- Is there a pet you can adopt to enliven your space?

At Work: Look around the space you spend time in. Dust and wipe down all surfaces.

- Clear old project files and notes from your desk, file cabinets, and those stacks on the floor. Shred any papers that have electronic copies or that you haven't needed or looked for a determined length of time.
- Delete emails from your mail server, old files off the computer, and contacts of those who you no longer even remember who they are.
- Replace the dead plants forgotten in the corner and old pictures or objects that do not reflect your healthy lifestyle and ambitions now.
- Scan any room and notice how the 'stuff' around you makes you feel. You may be so used to the clutter and state of things that you don't even realize it is affecting your body, health, and emotions. Brainstorm ways to clean, clear, and release that stagnant energy from the area.

- If you have work-related travel, always bring something with you or enjoy a routine that will keep your emotions and energy normal.
- Healing spaces can extend to choosing a vacation spot. Choose your time away with thoughts of how it will affect your emotions, energy, and ability to enjoy it. Taking a trip to Disney World and Epcot can be exhausting and full of anxiety for some but exciting and invigorating for others. Just being out of your routine is stressful for most people, so make it as comfortable and healing as possible.

Creating your healing spaces is about creating an environment that supports your healing. It is a way to ensure that you are including comfortable, holistic environments to reduce the strains and stresses of your daily life.

PRINCIPLE 17

MAKE IT SIMPLE

"Simplicity is the final achievement."

—FREDRIC CHOPIN

During the twenty or so years that my children were growing up, the whirlwind of activity never stopped. My days consistently included taking care of four children (in three different schools at times), owning our own business, attending sports events, volunteer work, and me working an additional outside job. The schedules and complexity of it all often took its toll not only on my energy but my brain capacity, as well. As I struggled to balance all the demands of work and family while keeping myself healthy, I became aware of how just simplifying and identifying the basics of everything I had to accomplish in the day was an important factor in staying ahead of the game. Later in life, after I was divorced and the kids were raised, I felt a new set of pressures and demands as I learned to support myself and identify with new roles as a mom of adult kids, grandma, and girlfriend. Again, the worries, thoughts, and schedules in my head seemed to never stop. At one point, seeing that my symptoms were worsening, I had to take a step back and look at not only what was really important for me to spend my time on, but to see how I could simplify my life to get rid of some of that constant barrage of thoughts and emotions.

Our modern lives have become unbelievably complex and are so packed with constant demands that it's no wonder we juggle a whirlwind of thoughts, actions, and emotions each day. Some days our minds feel like a browser with too many open tabs, each representing something we're trying to keep up with. The body becomes stuck in a fight-or-flight stress response, creating anxiety which disrupts and does not help the body's healing processes. Energy becomes diverted from healthy cell repair and production to being used by those fearful survival anxiety-driven stresses.

Often, the diagnosis of a disease itself is the wake-up call to slow down, and you are literally forced to simplify and focus. But focusing only on the illness or simplifying due to restrictions is not where you want to remain. Simplifying our lives can be a powerful tool in health management by reducing mental and physical clutter to allow your body and mind to focus on healing.

This does not need to mean doing without or even with less. It does mean that you determine what is important in the big picture for yourself, your loved ones, and the overall health outcome you are striving for. It is advantageous to keep your focus on developing your healing habits to keep the mind clutter and random thoughts in an organized state. By focusing thoughts and actions on just the big pieces, the smaller minute details that cause worry and anxiety will be kept at bay.

□ □ □

COMPLEXITY OF OUR MODERN LIFE

It is important to identify some of the areas to be aware of in your daily life that you may or may not realize are causing complexity and overwhelm.

- Our smartphones, laptops, and social media keeping us constantly plugged in with notifications about news, emails, and messages, creating constant mini distractions that require us to think about and respond.
- You may be balancing multiple jobs and side projects like volunteer work, juggling family time, hobbies, exercise, and social obligations that are all pulling your attention in different directions.
- The internet and easy access to endless information can be empowering but also overwhelming. Constantly seeking and processing new information creates a situation where our minds are always 'ON' working to process and digest it all.
- You may feel pressured to work on yourself, whether it's fitness, mental health, or learning new skills, and that often means planning and tracking activities, setting goals, and comparing progress with others, adding more to your daily mental overwhelm.
- Financial worries are a common stressor, with budgeting to paying bills, managing loans, or saving for future goals and add an underlying stress to daily life.
- We make hundreds of decisions daily, from the seemingly trivial (like choosing what to say or eat) to the important (such as career moves).
- Staying connected with friends, supporting family, and keeping up with social events and celebrations can be fulfilling but also mentally and physically draining. We often think about loved ones, their needs, and how to support them, which adds another layer of thinking.
- Your illness is a constant physical and mental issue in your life, and fatigue and limitations can be a constant source of

frustration as well as the mental drain from the uncertainty and anxiety of the unknown.

A simpler lifestyle reduces stress by helping us focus on what's truly important, like healthy habits, restful sleep, and positive relationships. When we streamline our schedules, prioritize activities that nourish us, and remove unnecessary commitments and people who drain us of energy, our minds feel calmer, which can strengthen our immune systems, improve our mental health, and boost energy levels. Additionally, a simpler life encourages mindful decision-making about food, exercise, and relaxation, creating that nurturing environment for the body to repair itself. By intentionally eliminating stressors and distractions that create overwhelm, we create the space needed to heal.

◻ ◻ ◻

HEALING HABIT 17: KEEP IT FUN AND SIMPLE

Emotions to develop: Hopeful, Calm
Emotions to be aware of: Anxiety, Frustration, Overwhelm

Each chapter of our lives represents different activities, needs, and areas of focus. No matter what age we are, worries, schedules, and input are coming into our minds and bodies that need to be managed and organized. As you give yourself permission to develop and focus on your healing habits, simplifying your life comes naturally, but those same habits must be easy to implement. Do not let the idea of changing become a belief that you need to do more and do it better. Instead, look at the ways to turn 'OFF' the chatter and make developing habits fun.

- **Set Boundaries on Screen Time**: Limit social media or news-checking to specific times and make a habit of *not* looking at your phone or emails while doing something else.
- **Create a Short To-Do List**: Rather than a long list of everything you need to do in the next week, stick to a daily list of three to five essential tasks. Focus on quality over quantity to avoid feeling overwhelmed and to feel a sense of accomplishment. As the list is completed, reward yourself and then list another three to five tasks if you still have time left in your day. Make sure that there is something that makes you smile at the top of each list. Find ways to add some fun to any task—dance, sing, recite poetry, or picture yourself as superwoman.
- **Schedule 'No Commitment' Days**: Designate a day each week with no planned activities. Use this time to rest, explore hobbies, or recharge without any demands on your time.
- **Practice Daily Decluttering**: Spend five to ten minutes each day organizing a small area, like your workspace, bedroom, or kitchen counter. This habit reduces visual and mental clutter, helping you feel more focused.
- **Adopt the 'One In, One Out' Rule**: Whenever you buy something new, let go of a similar item. This keeps possessions from piling up and helps maintain a balanced, clutter-free healing space environment.
- **Plan Weekly Meals**: Pre-plan and pre-shop for meals to save time and reduce decision fatigue. This habit also makes you stick to your healthier diet since you're less likely to opt for last-minute fast food. Engage family members, if possible, to include some quality time during meal prep.
- **Mindful moments**: Spend a few minutes each morning and evening reflecting on your day and focusing on what made

you smile or was fun. If there is nothing coming up for you, make sure you add that to tomorrow's list.

Implementing these simplifying habits into your life will reach throughout each of the healing principles you are learning here. Many times, the complexity of our days and the voice in our head becomes so loud that we do not even realize or appreciate the moment we are in, let alone recognize the life we are leading. Simplify life's demands, reduce stress, and create space for what's meaningful.

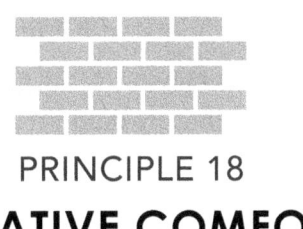

PRINCIPLE 18
CREATIVE COMFORT

"I am seeking. I am striving. I am in it with all my heart."
−VINCENT VAN GOGH

Often, we participate in activities that bring us comfort without realizing the significance. Cooking, baking, and preserving food are some of those activities for me. The habit developed in part to eat the freshest foods possible and stay away from fast foods, but also to carry on a tradition of preserving foods handed down from my grandmothers. The kitchen was primarily my domain, and even with a full schedule, I usually never minded taking the time to put together a meal or bake fresh desserts. It was comforting and a creative way for me to unwind that, at the time, I took for granted. This became evident when, later in life, I found myself in a relationship that focused on going out to eat most every night after coming home from work. While I appreciated the gesture of being taken out, I was frustrated that I couldn't just cook us a meal and relax. I found that the comfort of preparing the meal was an important way to soothe my stress of the day and provide needed relaxation.

You may not be one to describe cooking dinner or canning tomatoes as your number one downtime activity, but we each have things we do that make us feel safe, where we can relax our minds and calm our nerves. It is, in essence, a hug we give ourselves. Our busy, productivity-driven modern lives typically hold very little time for doing the things we enjoy. By intentionally choosing to include activities that bring us comfort, it supports not only our emotions but our physical body, as well, by boosting the immune system. It cultivates a needed environment that shifts us from that stressful 'fight or flight' mode into 'rest and repair' for our bodies.

Much of our daily life can be spent in the frustration of dealing with painful symptoms and fear of the unknown when we have a chronic illness. Comfort can come from familiar routines and simple pleasures that not only nurture our bodies but also soothe our minds, allowing us to unwind from the stresses of the day. Our bodies react to what the mind is feeling, and choosing to indulge in activities that bring balance, enjoyment and calmness to our personal world will only enhance the healing process.

◻◻◻

THE ARTIST WITHIN

Creativity is a trait that has often been squashed in our overly productive, driven society. Creative endeavors establish order in our lives, offering an outlet for self-expression and, more importantly, a means to process our emotions. Whether it's cooking, painting, writing, or crafting, engaging in creative activities provides a structured way to channel thoughts and feelings.

The process of creation can help you make sense of your experiences, turning chaos into clarity, fear into courage, and helplessness into strength and empowerment. As you immerse yourself in creative endeavors, you can find a rhythm that brings balance to your life, allowing you to step away from stress and focus on what matters most.

Combining cozy, comforting experiences with creative pursuits enhances your sense of well-being and fosters a deeper connection to yourself. When you take the time to engage in activities that bring you joy while providing downtime, you cultivate an environment that reduces stress and invites healing. Engaging in easy cozy rituals can evoke nostalgia, transporting you back to cherished moments, or they can support a daily chore that provides strength for your family. The cozy moments and creative pleasures you embrace are not just indulgences; they are essential habits that help to set your world in order, both nurturing your spirit and grounding you in the present. These habits can create calm within and a sense of purpose when nothing else can, adding comforting energy to nurture your sense of well-being and joy. These feel-good activities are habits that should be so ingrained that it is hard to live without them; they are your metaphoric comfort foods.

□ □ □

HEALING HABIT 18: CUDDLE UP WITH YOUR CREATIVE SIDE

Emotions to develop: Calmness
Emotions to be aware of: Imposter Syndrome, Judgement

We all can identify with having a creative pleasure or two that makes our hearts sing or helps set our world right when things seem anything but. These can be some of the want-to-dos or the lifestyle enhancers you previously identified, or maybe some of the routines you already have. These are the habits that allow you to put your phone down and your emails on hold and delve into another world. Remember, these are the activities you turn to each time a hug is needed.

- Identify something you really enjoy doing just for the fun of it, something that speaks to your heart. These activities are usually the ones that you lose yourself in and can spend hours doing without noticing the time flying by. How can you work these into your day?

Some new ideas can be:

- Light a fire or candle and journal by the soft natural light.
- Wrap up in a blanket and read a book, indulging in the escape.
- Engage in handmade crafts or gardening. Activities you enjoy to keep your hands busy can provide a sense of purpose, warmth, and relaxation. Knit a scarf, tie fishing flies, make seasonal decorations or gifts for others.
- Cooking and baking bring warmth and provide a sense of taking care of yourself and others. Experiment with new recipes or bake some of Grandma's sugar cookies.
- Create a cozy drink ritual with teas, hot cocoa, or spiced cider. Gather some cute mugs, unique blends, and maybe a sprinkle of spices, and enjoy a calming drink. Incorporating a healing tea blend can double the effects.
- Writing letters or handmade cards for friends and family offers a nostalgic, heartwarming feeling. Take yourself away from the computer and digital age for a bit.
- Curate playlists with soft, mellow tunes that give you a sense of warmth. You can enjoy them while doing other cozy activities or simply curl up and listen.
- Indulge in a candlelit bath. The advertising slogan for Calgon bath salts years ago of, "Calgon, take me away" no doubt sold

millions with its popularity. Every woman in America wanted to melt into a hot bath of fragrant salts and let the stresses melt away. Treat yourself with some candlelight and quiet.

Options in this category of habits to create are limitless and can support your peace and healing, providing you with a place to cozy up in to take care of you when needed.

◻ ◻ ◻

"There is no charm equal to tenderness of heart."

—JANE AUSTEN

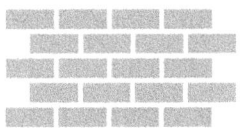

PRINCIPLE 19
REFLECT AND EVALUATE

Life is about constantly starting over, each moment of every day, and what a blessing that is!

I was a business manager at a Boy Scout camp for several years. Each Sunday before the new scout troops came in for the next week, the program director assembled the staff and there was an evaluation of the prior week to address any changes needed or situations to improve. We were also made aware of any upcoming issues and set goals for the coming week. It was the age of VCR tapes and, for those old enough to remember, there was a process to go through to be able to start the tape over again. STOP, REWIND, PLAY. This became our staff mantra, and we developed creative ways (songs, skits, raps, stories, etc.) to reset our minds and bodies for the upcoming week. It was so effective, I will still recite "Stop, Rewind, Play" to myself when faced with an everyday setback, a flare-up, or even knowing of a stressful situation coming up.

Our lives can change on a moment's notice, and rarely do things go along smoothly for very long. On the flip side, when we're feeling better, we often slip back into bad habits without giving them much thought. There is a power in awareness (STOP), evaluation (REWIND), and improved action (PLAY) that can get us through what life throws at us and keep us on our chosen path to well-being.

Managing your illness is a lifelong process and will take an everyday effort to first develop and then maintain your healthy habits. It is advantageous to create a routine evaluation and to take stock, reassess your lifestyle choices, and prepare for any future events. Situations and circumstances are in continual movement, and what may have worked for you last year or even last month may not be working for you today.

Reflection is a key element in growth and self-awareness. It allows you to pause, assess, and recalibrate as needed. Through a habit of reflection, you can identify patterns, acknowledge your progress, and recognize areas that may need some improvement. This important practice also creates a bridge between where you started from, where you are now, and your future vision. Taking the time to reflect, you will also be able to determine the positive advances your new habits are making in your life, which not only gives clarity but will build resilience to maintaining your choices.

□□□

SOME THINGS WORK, SOME DON'T

Recognize the patterns of what is working and what isn't, and don't be afraid to make changes as needed. You may need to develop new habits or tweak some of the old ones. Give yourself permission to adjust without guilt or self-judgment.

For example, medications can unexpectedly lose their effectiveness, or your lifestyle choices may become overwhelming. You might have moved from a fulfilling career to owning your own business or discovered that working for a nonprofit brings you greater joy. Perhaps the easygoing volunteer group you once loved now demands more of your time and energy, leaving you feeling overwhelmed and stressed. The juicing regimen that once boosted your health might suddenly start causing discomfort. All can be pivotable moments where a good evaluation can help identify a needed 180-degree turn.

Reflection can also be used to see the positive changes you have made and how your health has improved. Stop to notice your achievements, pat yourself on the back, and take your bows.

Use the habits of reflection and evaluation to quickly assess whether your lifestyle choices are working for or against your healing. This will provide you with the ability to quickly pivot if needed. Our goal is to create a lifestyle through habits that take care of you. Evaluation is the tool that leads us to circle back on the previous principles. It is always the right time to make some changes.

Having sight without insight is worse than not seeing the true potential of what lies ahead.

◻ ◻ ◻

HEALING HABIT 19: STOP, REWIND, PLAY

Emotions to develop: Hopefulness, Eagerness
Emotions to be aware of: Stagnant, Stuck

No matter how you are feeling in your health journey, it is important to reflect and evaluate. A good evaluation begins with seeing the big picture of what your health looks like. Does it look great, okay, but could it be better, or not as happy and healthy as I could be? If you are beginning to have symptoms again after a remission, take quick action to determine what the root cause is and then implement a quick solution. If you feel better than you have, take time to acknowledge it and identify the reasons. Taking the time to reflect is an intentional action that prevents you from falling into a 'wait and see' attitude, possibly to ignore the symptoms or resist changing your habits, and it will most likely defeat any previous efforts and progress you have made.

- Make a habit of setting aside an hour or so each month to reflect and evaluate your life, focusing specifically on how you feel. Go through the previous principles and touch on each of them to reassess where you are today. Some questions to ask yourself may be:

    Have you been lazy or successful about keeping most of the toxins out of your life?

    Are you eating more whole, nutritious foods than processed?

    Have you been getting the proper amount of rest you need?

    How are you spending your time? Are you including enough 'want-to-dos?' Have you eliminated some of the 'have-to-dos?' Are you feeling good about those decisions?

    Is there just one thing you've been doing you could change to make things better?

    Are the boundaries you set still relevant?

    Is there a life enhancer you recently heard of you that want to try out?

    Are you celebrating your successes?

    Is there something you need to say no to when asked again?

    Is there something you need to say yes to?

Does your space need a good cleaning or clutter clearing?

Are you taking enough time for your creative pursuits?

Carve out at least fifteen minutes each day to just be with your thoughts and tune-in. This can be while meditating outside or while you prepare for bed. Be conscious of you and how your life and body is feeling. Many times, this process alone will give valuable insight into making those quick pivots.

What are you grateful for, and what is going right?

How did you react to people today?

How do you feel physically? Better or worse than last week?

How do you feel mentally?

Are you feeling fulfilled by activities and successes today or frustrated and angry?

Was it a good day? How can you incorporate those peaceful feelings?

Was it a frustrating day? What parts were tense? How can you let go of those feelings and replace them with gratitude?

Are you happy overall and at peace or worried and just hanging on by your fingertips?

It is human nature to stay on the path of least resistance and to get stuck in outdated feelings, thoughts, and habits. You need to take the time to reflect and evaluate and then re-evaluate your lifestyle and pivot as often as necessary. Implementing these healing principles is not a once and done process.

STOP, REWIND & REPLAY
REFLECTION TIME

I feel better when:

My Happy Places:

Not doing this again:

Areas to work on:

Boundaries I have maintained!

I am proud of myself for:

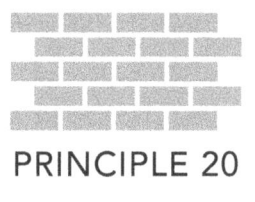

PRINCIPLE 20
PUT A SMILE ON IT

> *"The happiness of your life depends upon the quality of your thoughts."*
>
> –MARCUS AURELIUS (MEDITATIONS, C. 170—180 AD)

I have been accused of being overly optimistic and berated for smiling in the face of adversity. It's true; I have often smiled in situations that seem dire at best, giving the impression that I don't care or that I am not taking the situation seriously, sometimes frustrating those around me. It is not as it seems. I believe that seeing a situation with amusement takes the sting out of it and puts whatever the issue is into perspective. Smiling through adversity gives you power, it stops the dark from getting in, and it keeps your focus on the bigger picture. This has become my foundation for not only managing symptoms of disease but my life in general. Dealing with a chronic illness has a lot of bad moments, and it is not that I don't take my situation seriously—it means I don't stay in that place. While I do have my 'aahh, sh*t' moments, my 'd*mn this disease' days, and my well h*ll weeks, they do not define my life.

There seems to be a cultural stigma around being happy that arises from societal norms and expectations that view joy with skepticism or even disdain. If you are someone who expresses joy or optimism, especially in challenging circumstances, you can be judged as naive, insincere, or dismissive of others' struggles. This can often discourage you from openly celebrating achievements and expressing happiness or lead to feelings of guilt or shame for feeling happy in light of your troubles. In professional settings, happiness can be perceived as a lack of seriousness or commitment. It is, to say the least, unfair and assuming but there nonetheless.

You may have experienced this stigma in dealing with your illness, where you may have had your struggles dismissed or invalidated if you appear happy. You may have heard more than once, "You don't look or act sick." This can obviously pressure you to downplay your positive emotions and becomes an issue when you hold others shame or guilt or even the joy inside your body. When faced with this stigma, it is best to remember that how you perceive your life and the emotions you carry within are your business.

Letting this judgement of being happy and the inability to express joy land in your body and affect your life is one of the precursors of illness and a root cause that needs addressed. The authenticity of being happy and feeling positive emotions needs to be included in your identity. If you are happy in mind and heart, your body is happy physically. Embrace and normalize happiness as a valid and valuable emotion—do not settle for moderation and conformity.

□□□

HAPPY AS A LARK

Chronic illnesses are not a picnic by anyone's definition, but you can put whatever it is into perspective and see the moment with amusement, even if it is not pleasant. This is best achieved when you acknowledge the blessings in your life, focus on what's going well, and respond with gratitude. The choice is always yours of whether you see the silver lining or stay stuck scowling in the storm clouds. Let those happy emotions out and never settle for that negative, stressful conformity. If you can focus on being happy and appreciate the positives, you will find that controlling your illness and its symptoms is possible. Look for those glimmers in your life.

In our mission to listen to the body, if you can adopt a habit of a cheerful attitude and amusement, it is easier to hear what your body is telling you and react accordingly. What you are doing and feeling has, without a doubt, an effect on your health, good, bad, or otherwise, and it is easier to listen with a smile.

Humor and laughter do play essential roles in managing chronic illnesses. Laughter boosts immune function, reduces stress, and improves heart health, is highly contagious, and helps create a positive healing environment. That is certainly something to smile about.

> *"Out beyond ideas of wrong doing and right doing, there is a field. I'll meet you there...."*
>
> —RUMI

HEALING HABIT 20: DON'T WORRY, BE HAPPY

Developing a habit of smiling on the inside involves consistently choosing perspectives and actions that nurture joy and happiness regardless of external circumstances. Practicing mindfulness and gratitude helps you stay in the moment, not worrying about the past or future. Surrounding yourself with positive influences in your environment reinforces a mindset that all is well. Do the things that make your body smile and release those endorphins. Several of these suggestions have already been mentioned but are worth repeating.

- Focus on the positives in your life by practicing gratitude. Writing down or just acknowledging thanks and small wins can shift your mindset to appreciation and joy.
- Surround yourself with uplifting people who provide encouragement and understanding to build a strong support system, reminding you that you are not alone and who you can smile with.
- Make it a habit to stop, look around, and smile at something or someone several times throughout your day. Laugh at yourself and the predicaments you get yourself into.
- Focus on small victories and celebrate your wins each day. Completing a task, enjoying a meal, or finding a moment of calm are all achievements to remind you of your resilience and progress.
- Engage in creative activities like painting, writing, or music to channel your thoughts positively and bring out that inner smile.

- Participate in endorphin-releasing activities that can boost your mood when you are feeling down like playing sports, getting out in the sunlight, laughing, and acts of kindness.
- Develop a morning affirmation habit by starting your day with a positive affirmation such as, "I am strong, and I will face today with courage," and a smile.
- Choose a meaningful trinket to keep with you or someplace you frequent that reminds you to smile. This can be anything from a favorite smooth crystal to keep in your pocket to a picture on your visor in your car, a piece of jewelry or small statue next to your bed. Each time you notice your special trinket smile!

There will always be the option of feeling miserable for years or deciding to quickly shake it off with positive action, putting a smile back on your face and in your heart. If you are not all you want to be, then do what you need to do to grow. If you are sick and tired of being sick and tired, take the leap of faith to follow a new path. Smiling through adversity is a good habit to achieve your desired destination.

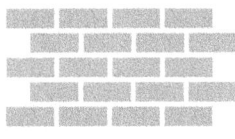

CONCLUSION
THRIVING NOT JUST SURVIVING

The #1 habit to develop is to take care of you.

Being diagnosed with and living daily with a chronic disease is not easy and will forever change the trajectory of the life you have lived until now. But that does not need to be the end of the story. By seeing a diagnosed disease not as a death sentence but a blessing in disguise, you can look with a different perspective at your life. *you* have the blessing of your body telling you that your lifestyle habits (how the way you live affects your body) could be better, and with some effort, it will show you what the cause and solution could be.

You need to develop the belief and awareness that your body innately knows how to be healthy and can heal itself if given the right environment and support. It is within your power to provide that healing environment. Give yourself permission when needed, support when necessary, and ideas to think about alongside the conventional medical treatment box. Everyone on the planet has something that is amiss with their health; most just don't acknowledge it or know it yet.

You can decide how sick you want to be— and you can help your body heal itself.

You can be a key player in your health, and it is in your best interest to take responsibility and take on the executive director's role. I encourage you to be a top-level executive; the architect embodying not only the creative designer but also the visionary, the builder, the collaborator, the planner, and the supervisor of your life. Manage your health personally and like your life depends on it—because it does!

Chronic illnesses can be managed by reducing symptoms and allowing space for your body to heal. This book is about what 'managing' your disease takes. It is about what it means to release damaging habits to create space for new healing habits. It is about how to embody those habits into a healing lifestyle. It is about how to create an identity that sees you as a healthy person supporting and taking responsibility to help your body heal itself. It is to remind you of the power you have over your life to be anything you want to be, and that includes being healthy and happy.

The twenty principles and healing habits that have been presented here are a foundation for you to begin to define what and how you want your life to look. They are the foundational behaviors that you can use as your operating manual. There are no outlandish or new concepts, just a reminder of how the way we live and the things we do in our modern life affect our physical, emotional, and spiritual bodies. Take and use what is most relevant to your situation.

Conventional medicine has its place in chronic illness and disease management, and is very much needed to diagnose and treat acute symptoms, begin reversing inflammation, or repair damage. Unfortunately, that same conventional medicine makes us believe we have no choice but to continue to only follow that standard of care, which many have found is not the best way to manage a disease over time.

It simply is not sustainable, nor does it promote real healing in the body, which is ultimately needed to reduce symptoms.

I have come across people who feel that their chronic illness is justified, that this is the cross they bear or that fate has handed them this particular struggle to maneuver forever. While that may indeed have credence, it is also just as credible to believe that you have unknowingly led a life that, due to toxins and other contributing factors, has given cause to the dis-ease and eventual illness in your body. There is great power in believing what has been done can be undone; that everything in your life has developed over time, and over time can be set right.

There is a mass turning point beginning to take shape in our society that is moving toward more self-directed preventative health care and a more spiritual, energetic, and loving connection with our own physical bodies. We have begun to look for answers as we become more responsible for our lifestyles and the associated chronic illnesses our bodies have inevitably developed. It has become a Catch-22; a frustrating dilemma of balancing disease (health) management between what is conventional and convenient against addressing what caused the illness and taking responsibility to reduce stresses in the body.

If you are ready to redefine your disease management into health management and ready to see a different way to address your symptoms and diagnosis, try something outside the norm. These healing habits can be your foundation.

□□□

LIFE BEYOND ILLNESS

These are practices that each and every one of us can accomplish and incorporate into our daily lives. There are stories from every part of the globe of those who have cured their own stage 4 cancers, type 2 diabetes, Crohn's disease, fibromyalgia, multiple sclerosis, and so many more chronic illnesses. There are stories of such triumph that it inspired new research careers in alternative healing, energy work, and clean foods. Many of these patients began just where you are now. Their pain, loss, and suffering pushed them into making a choice to help themselves overcome their circumstances and not succumb to the norm.

You should, in every circumstance, have the choice to take control of your own health without ever feeling like the victim of your disease. You can no longer be reliant or confident in living with the mass-produced lifestyle inherited from society, government, and big pharma. You need to take back your own body, mind, and soul and make your life worth living in a healthy, more enjoyable way.

I have found that when adverse things do come around, giving yourself the grace to see beyond immediate circumstances is all about belief. Believing you have the power within you, believing your body is a living organism that desires optimal functioning, believing that there is enough information available, believing that you have control over your own health.

Life itself is about the ups and downs, the highs and lows, the 'ecstatic' and 'please God help me' moments; none of us escape that reality. But if you so choose, you can create your new normal, and rather than continuing to live a life that supports illness, instead live one that supports your body to heal itself. It is my hope that by telling my story as a colleague and friend, you can see yourself as someone who can begin to take care of yourself and have great success doing it.

To your health.

> **Life does not stand still, and each day we are pushed to become the future selves we didn't know we could become**

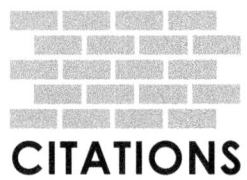

CITATIONS

CLEAR, J. (2018). *Atomic habits*. Avery.
Clear, Ja. (n.d.). How to Master the Art of Continuous Improvement by James Clear . *Continuous Improvement: How It Works and How to Master It*.

Clear, Ja. (n.d.). *How to Change Your Beliefs and Stick to Your Goals for Good*.

Mee, B. (2011). *We bought a zoo*. 20th Century Fox.

Imai, M. (2024, September 24). *What is KaizenTM*. Meaning Of Kaizen.

Canfield, J., & Switzer, J. (2012). *Success principles*. HarperCollins Christian Publishing.

Renck, R. (2016). *Live Healthy with Crohn's disease: 13 aspects to managing your disease to live a symptom-free life*. Balboa Press, a division of Hay House.

Photo Credit by Suzie Bauer
Portrait photographer
@photographybysooz

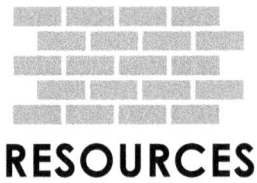

RESOURCES

It would be impossible to note all the resources and knowledge I have internalized during my lifetime—most is personal experience, but I have profoundly benefited from the many articles, stories, and books selflessly written by others sharing their wisdom over the years. The following are some of the more influential books and resources that I have found to be helpful in my journey of developing strength within myself and eventually healing habits. In addition to the Citations listed I would include the following as instrumental in my lifelong journey.

Heal Breast Cancer Naturally by Dr. Veronique Desaulniers-Chomniak. TCK Publishing. (2016).

Turtle Wisdom: Coming Home to Yourself by Donna Denomme. Your Wisdom Story Publishing (2023).
This trusted guide for living a happy, authentic life uplifts you on a bad day, reminds you of your inherent worth in moments of self-doubt, and gives you a boost no matter what. Voted "Industry Choice" and "Book of the Year" 2024 by Donna Denomme.

8 Keys to Wholeness: Tools for Hope-Filled Healing by Donna Denomme. Inlightened Source Publishing (2014).

Utilizing the ancient chakra system as a container for our wounding, we find powerful ways to release what no longer serves us. We cultivate enduring strength and unbeatable resilience, as we stretch into our heart's desires and soul's longings to realize our greatest soul expression.

Ask And It Is Given—Part I and Part II
by Abraham & Esther and Jerry Hicks. Hay House Publishing (2005).

Unlock the Secret Messages of Your Body!: A 28-Day Jump-Start Program for Radiant Health and Glorious Vitality by Denise Linn. Hay House Publishing (2011)

Follow the Author at www.rebeccarenck.com

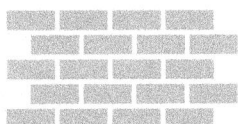

ACKNOWLEDGMENTS

Like many authors, turning thoughts into a readable, published book only happens with much encouragement and a great deal of support. I am no exception. I did not have a burning desire to be a writer, but I knew I had a message to share—one that could encourage and empower others. I have achieved more than I ever imagined, discovering my voice and an unexpected passion for writing. This journey has given me a new purpose, career, friendships, and confidence, all supported by the incredible encouragement of my editing and production team. This book would not have come to fruition without them.

I am deeply grateful for the doctors, nurses, parents, alternative health practitioners, and public figures who are standing up for our health rights and bringing attention to the need for change in the current healthcare system. Their dedication has paved the way for functional medicine clinics and alternative treatment centers, making holistic medicine a part of everyday conversations and in many cases the first choice for care. I am especially grateful for the dedication and perseverance of alternative care practitioners, herbalists, nutritionists, and energy workers whose work has proven that supporting the body's natural healing process delivers real results. They have promoted an amazing transformation into preventive and sustainable healthcare.

I appreciate my daughters and sister for embracing both holistic and conventional medicine, showing that each has value. Their willingness to be pioneers in their chosen fields and practices has given me the confidence to share my journey and speak out on the importance of listening to our bodies and making informed health decisions.

I am humbled and filled with gratitude for each reader who has picked up *Healing Habits* with an open heart and a willingness to embrace change in their own lives. It takes courage to step outside familiar routines; to embrace and explore a new perspective on health and healing. Your commitment to learning, growing, and reclaiming your personal well-being is inspiring. Thank you for allowing me to be part of your journey—I honor your dedication to creating a healthier, more empowered life.

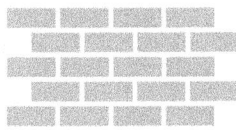

ABOUT THE AUTHOR

At thirty years old, Rebecca was diagnosed with acute Crohn's disease. With four young children to raise and a lifetime of experiences she had yet to live, she chose *not* to let this diagnosis and disease rule her life. In short, she decided how sick she wanted to be and how she wanted her life to look.

She has become a strong believer in our own personal healing power. By focusing on self-development, listening to her body, reducing toxins, and practicing holistic remedies, she created a roadmap of principles and healing habits that allowed her to help the body to heal itself. Today, the disease still has its minor days, but she can quickly get back to a state of wellness using these same principles and by refining her habits. Looking back on the daily choices made, she is proud of her efforts and believes that everyone can have the same healthy outcome with the correct mindset and tools at their disposal.

Rebecca is not a medical doctor and would never profess to be but has thirty plus years of experience in managing her Crohn's disease and a breast cancer diagnosis with minimal medical intervention and holistic practices. As a caretaker, she has been a strong advocate for those with chronic illnesses. By sharing her own journey, she offers support and encouragement, showing that even small changes can help the body heal itself. She is passionate in her grounded, no-nonsense approach in the belief that conventional medicine is not our only option when managing a disease and its symptoms and is passionate about sharing the foundation to developing the habits that can help your body heal itself.

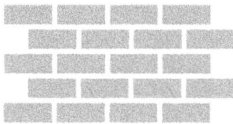

FREE OFFERS

- Get A Bonus Chapter on *How to Apply These Ideas as a Caretaker*. This extra Chapter can be requested and downloaded by sending an email to rebecca@rebeccarenck.com
- Join the Healing Habits newsletter at www.healinghabitsbook.com